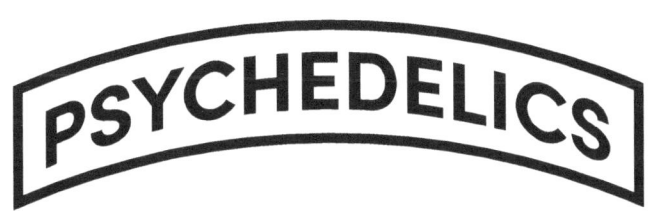

THE VETERAN'S FIELD MANUAL

Healing PTSD and trauma through psychedelic and MDMA therapy

JESSE GOULD

Army Ranger,
Heroic Hearts Project Founder

with **ELAINE MARSHALL**

THE VETERAN'S FIELD MANUAL FOR PSYCHEDELICS: HEALING PTSD
AND TRAUMA THROUGH PSYCHEDELIC AND MDMA THERAPY
by Jesse Gould with Elaine Marshall

ISBN: 979-8-9925509-0-0

To my beautiful wife, Ana — whose pure love, patience, and belief in me have carried me through every storm.

To the Heroic Hearts team — the family that turned vision into reality.

And to all the veterans still fighting — for healing, for peace, for one another — this book is for you.

— Jesse

I dedicate this book to John E. Lamphear, Ph.D., Professor Emeritus of African and Military History at the University of Texas. Your integrity and impeccable standards opened my eyes to a new world, including within myself.

And to Glenn, for helping me find my way through, spoonful by spoonful.

— Elaine

CONTENTS

FOREWORD

As a Marine, I learned early on in my career that you never leave a fellow warrior behind. That principle doesn't end when a veteran returns home, yet too many of our brothers and sisters come back from service only to face internal battles no one prepared them for. Every day, we lose more veterans to suicide. That is not acceptable, and it should weigh heavily on all of us. Behind each number is a name, a family, a story cut short. These were men and women who once carried our nation's burdens, and their loss is a reminder of the cost of inaction. We owe them better.

This book confronts the reality that too many of our veterans come home to a system that cannot meet their needs. But more importantly, it points to a way forward. It reflects the strength of veterans who refuse to give up, who are willing to explore new paths to healing when the old ones have failed.

What you'll find here is not theory. It's the lived experience of men and women who know the cost of service, and who are leading once again by example. They are showing us that healing is possible, that hope can return, and that veterans themselves are often the strongest advocates for the care they need.

The Veteran's Field Manual for Psychedelics is exactly what the title suggests: a guide written by and for those still in the fight. It is a resource, a compass, and in many cases, a lifeline. My hope is that it will help veterans reclaim their health, restore their families, and remind our country of the duty we share to those who served.

Semper Fi,

Major General Paul Kennedy USMC (Ret.)
Board Member, Heroic Hearts Project

CHAPTER 1

FROM WALL STREET TO THE WAR ZONE TO HEALING

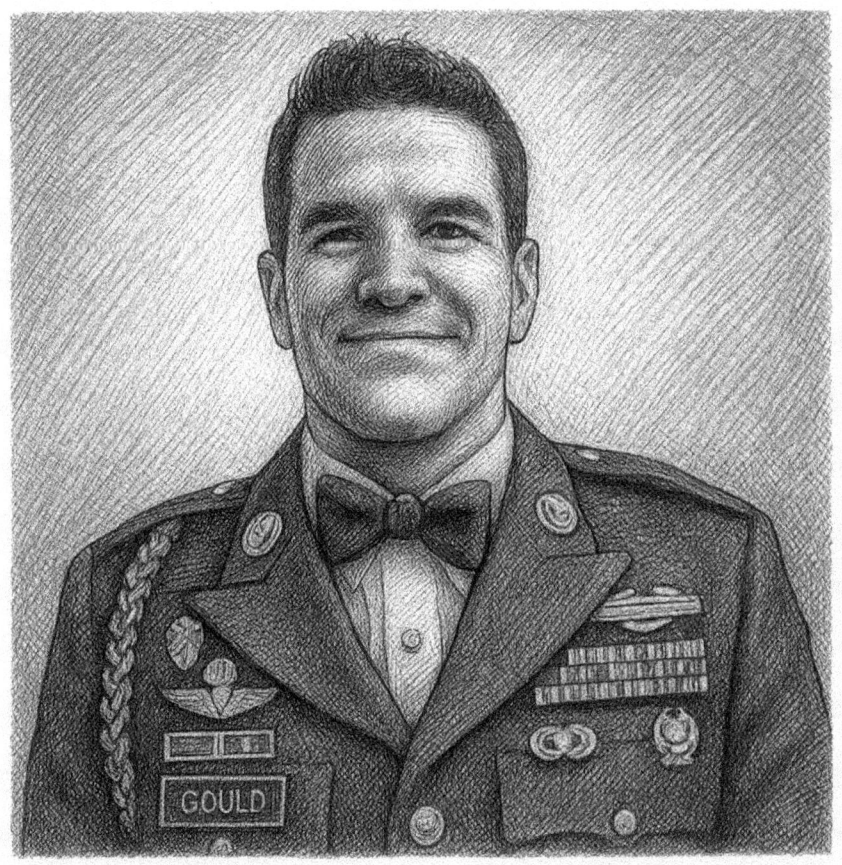

Jesse Gould, Army Ranger Veteran and founder of Heroic Hearts Project

I couldn't believe it was happening again, only it was worse than the previous two nights. A tornado ripped through my mind, tearing down buildings, splintering power lines, and hurling cows and cars into a pitch-black sky. The jungle heat pressed down like a vice, grinding my body through an invisible machine while I convulsed over a bucket, retching with merciless force.

I'd faced major challenges before: watching the economy implode from a Wall Street office in 2008, the relentless mud of infantry training, the starvation of Ranger school, and being deployed into the chaos of the United States' war on the Taliban in Afghanistan, where I was sent unprepared to lead and left with brain injuries and scars. As my mental health worsened back in New York City, I took to aimlessly wandering the streets at night and sleeping outside even though I had a warm home, just trying to feel something again.

But none of it came close to this night in the Peruvian jungle. My mind was fracturing. I was watching myself go insane. All I could do was survive each breath, one second at a time. But each second stretched into an eternity, screaming through my head like an air-raid siren, shattering me into a thousand sharp pieces.

And yet, somehow, to my astonishment, the following day I found myself writing a letter of apology to my parents as a dark certainty settled into me. Facing the prospect of repeating the ordeal again that night, I threw in the towel. My psyche would not survive another night. "I want to thank you for everything and apologize for what I'm about to do," I wrote. "I don't know if this will drive me insane, but I have to try—it feels like the only way left to fix myself. I know how much worry I've already caused, and I hate that. But I couldn't keep living the way I have been. I've tried everything I could, and nothing worked. This is my last attempt to find some peace, even if it costs me my mind."

The fight beat out of me, I resigned myself to the third evening, and shuffled to the *maloca* as if to my execution. I forced down the small cup of foul brew, grimaced at the taste, and lay back on my mat. Predictably, the tornado came rushing back, outraged. I braced myself for the meat grinder. Only this time, without warning, a blueish-green hand gently reached into the sweltering vortex toward me. I met its grip and instantaneously found myself sitting on the golden sand of the sapphire-blue Caribbean, a cool breeze wafting over me as the waves quietly lapped. A stillness infused my body with tender motherly love. My mind startled. What just happened? What caused this? I instinctively struggled to analyze the experience. And, whoosh, the vortex sucked me back into the noise, pain, and confusion. I bounced back and forth between these two worlds for the rest of the evening. My inquisitive, analytical mind would pull me into the tornado one moment, where I'd remember the only way to return to the peaceful shoreline was to surrender to the chaos.

As the medicine wore off and dawn broke through the jungle canopy, I took stock of this newfound agency over my psyche. The medicine had blasted through the neurological barbed wire of my injured and PTSD-addled brain. Just a month earlier, I lay in my bed as I had most nights, unable to sleep and staring in yet another drunken stupor at the ceiling. In the weeks that followed that first ayahuasca experience, I marveled at the return of my cognition, the loosening of my hypervigilance, and my ability to socialize while stone-cold sober.

However, something kept jamming the gears of my newfound neurological liberation: the almost weekly emails and texts delivering the news that yet another fellow Army Ranger had taken their own life. Or they were back in rehab, had lost their job, were divorcing, or falling apart in some other way.

The realization fell on me with crushing clarity. Across America, veterans were drowning in the same cycles of darkness, nightmares, hypervigilance, and alcohol-numbed pain I had been trapped in. They weren't responding to the same treatments from the VA that I had been through. They were writing their own goodbye letters.

I had no resources, no connections, and no blueprint to follow. What I did have was the Rangers' creed etched into my soul: "Never shall I fail my comrades." This wasn't a choice. It was an obligation as binding as any military order…a homework assignment from the cosmos.

————From the Ivy League to the Army Rangers————

I didn't come from a military family. Quite the opposite. I grew up anxiously shuttling between my divorced parents' homes in two different states, and despite a modest economic background, I academically earned my way into Cornell University. There, studying economics and working across the street from the New York Stock Exchange, I had a front-row seat to the 2008 financial collapse. I watched people lose everything overnight—savings, homes, and identities—reaffirming my childhood experiences that security is an illusion.

Although I had a mind for numbers, I did not have a personality for Wall Street. Mathematics and Excel sheets are reassuringly transparent. The culture around them, however, was a labyrinth of social riddles, doublespeak, and ulterior motives. I'd watch people say one thing while meaning another and smile at ideas they'd later sabotage. I learned that merit was a convenient myth sold to outsiders, when in reality, socioeconomic status determined who prospered and who merely survived.

Young, restless, and disillusioned, I yearned for something my Ivy League education couldn't give me, a primal "initiation" that would test my mettle. The Lakotas' wilderness vision quests, the Australian Aborigines' six-month walkabout, and the Maasais' lion hunt were all survival challenges that marked the transition from childhood to adulthood. Going to college didn't scratch this ancient itch, and I feared being stuck in a purgatory between youth and adulthood.

Which is how I found my way into an Army recruiting office during the height of the Iraq and Afghanistan surges. While my degree qualified me for officer candidacy, I chose the enlisted path. I wanted to know what I was made of, not what I could command others to do, whereupon I encountered the first of many reality checks.

Basic training shattered any romantic notions I had about the military. Although I didn't come from wealth, the poverty I encountered struck me in its rawness. Many of my fellow recruits were high school dropouts from economically decimated rust-belt towns, were avoiding jail, or trying to escape some aspect of their former lives. They weren't bad people, but it was a stark, unglamorous glimpse into the many faces of military recruitment and a sharp contrast to the manicured quads of Cornell and the marble lobbies of Wall Street.

After finishing at the top of my basic training class, due to the needs of the Army, I was assigned as a Mortarman, one of the least desired roles, and the source of my future brain injury from countless blast exposures. Nevertheless, I pushed through Mortarman training, Airborne School, Ranger Selection, and deployment.

The Ranger Selection and Assessment Program wasn't training; it was systematic destruction and rebuilding. For eight weeks, I existed in a fog of starvation, sleep deprivation, and exposure to the relentless, suffocating heat of a Georgia summer. By the end, I had lost thirty pounds, my uniform hanging from my frame. But I had succeeded. While I didn't go through any epic Hollywood-style battle moments in Afghanistan, people around me were wounded

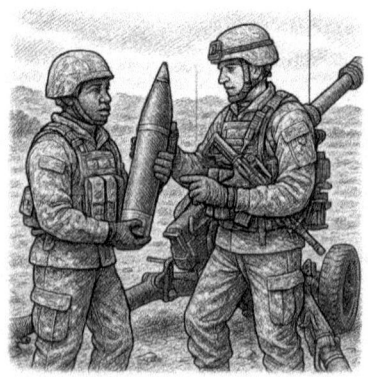

Mortarman training set the stage for brain injury that would exacerbate PTSD symptoms.

and killed. I survived a two-story fall from a collapsed roof, shock from live wires, mortar attacks, extreme temperatures, toxic dust, contaminated water, and the invisible toll of repeated blast exposures.

The slow unraveling after leaving the military

After leaving the military, I traveled through Europe and Southeast Asia, working odd jobs along the way. Beneath the excitement of travel and partying, I noticed a growing sense of anxiety and depression I couldn't explain.

Back in the U.S., I was rejected from job after job despite an impressive resume. I was broke, drinking heavily, and plagued by a profound sense of purposelessness. I finally landed a job in finance, but my nihilistic downward spiral continued. I engaged in consistently risky behaviors, such as walking through dangerous neighborhoods at night, sleeping on the streets, drinking before work, and moving through life with a "come at me" mentality. While high-functioning and not explicitly suicidal, I unconsciously hoped I'd stumble into a situation that would do the dirty work of taking my life for me.

I was unraveling but helpless to stop the descent, and needed a significant change.

Getting help at the VA

After a two-year wait, I was finally seen for a 45-minute assessment at the VA, where I was diagnosed with PTSD, spinal damage, and other injuries (brain injury was not assessed). I tried everything to improve, yet something remained fundamentally broken. My anxiety had graduated to intense panic attacks, and I doubled down on my drinking to manage the symptoms. I rejected psychiatric medications because I had seen them turn my friends into shells of their former selves. Eventually, I realized the VA wasn't able to help me and that if I wanted to get better, it was up to me to figure it out.

Around this time, I heard of psychedelics while listening to an Aubrey Marcus interview on Joe Rogan's podcast. I was dismissive of psychedelics as a treatment option, but because I had minored in Latin American studies and spent time living in Ecuador during college, the cultural and historical significance of ayahuasca caught my attention.

In late 2016, after researching and applying to a retreat center, quitting my job, and selling everything that didn't fit into a backpack, I departed for Peru to do ayahuasca.

Finding what I was searching for

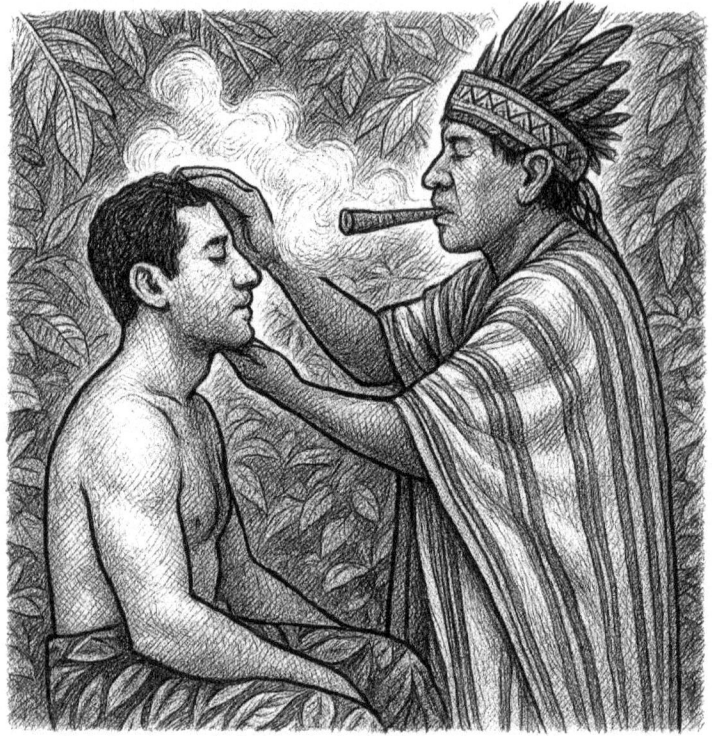

Ayahuasca pulled Gould out of a downward spiral, healed his brain injury, and inspired him to found Heroic Hearts Project

That fourth ayahuasca ceremony gave me what I'd been searching for: a sense of purpose and a reconnection with my warrior spirit of service and devotion.

It also helped me reconcile my lifelong struggle with the uncertainty and insecurity inherent in life.

"Trust yourself," a voice had said during that fourth journey. "You have the skills and determination to handle whatever comes your way."

———The role of TBIs in mental health crises———

The ayahuasca experience also shocked me as to how profound the symptoms from my undiagnosed traumatic brain injury (TBI) had become.

As a Mortarman, I'd experienced thousands of mortar explosions, rocket blasts, door breaches, and repeated concussive impacts from parachute jumps and falls, all of which had injured my brain.

Anxiety, depression, racing thoughts that wouldn't organize themselves, impulsive decisions I couldn't explain later, and a mind that would fixate on something one day and abandon it the next, had become the norm. I had attributed these symptoms to character flaws or PTSD, but now I understood they were caused by brain injury.

When my brain function returned after the ayahuasca retreat, that scattered, self-sabotaging state had been replaced by one of integration and purpose. A chilling thought emerged: how many of my brothers and sisters who had taken their own lives were spurred on by the symptoms of brain injury? How many were dismissed as having PTSD or depression when a brain injury was making coherent thought and emotional regulation nearly impossible?

————The birth of Heroic Hearts Project————

After the ayahuasca retreat, I landed in Guatapé, Colombia, a colorful lakeside town, and took a job at a motorcycle rental shop. It was a period of gentle self-discovery and integration. I still struggled with the pull of old patterns, but ayahuasca had opened a door where formerly only a wall had existed. I recognized that healing isn't a destination but an ongoing journey of constant recommitment.

When I began sharing my story, I was met with a surprising level of understanding. My parents saw the profound changes and were supportive. Fellow veterans responded with a military-like practicality: "If it works, it works."

I launched Heroic Hearts Project from a Colombian internet café on April 1, 2017. Short on money, but long on passion and purpose, I began spreading the word through online forums.

The right people appeared at pivotal moments, but building HHP was a relentless push, with progress coming in small increments.

A turning point came in 2018 with the publication of Michael Pollan's book *How to Change Your Mind*, which legitimized psychedelics for the mainstream. That same year, Johns Hopkins University opened its Psychedelic Research Center and the Multidisciplinary Association of Psychedelic Studies (MAPS) published promising results on MDMA-assisted therapy for PTSD.

Suddenly, HHP was at the forefront. We gained the attention of Dr. Bronner's, Silicon Valley tech donors, and other donors, which enabled us to evolve into an organization with occasional stipends and a small paid staff.

The work remains a steady march forward and as urgent today as when we began, with veteran suicide rates still tragically high and conventional treatments falling short for too many.

Today, running a nonprofit in the psychedelic space is its own spiritual practice. Constant funding uncertainty, working with trauma-affected veterans, and high workloads require me to continually work on strategies for self-care and balance.

That blue-green hand reaching through the chaos didn't just save me. It put me on a path to help my brothers and sisters in arms, fighting invisible battles with broken weapons, and learn how to save themselves. This work is now more my medicine than the one growing in the jungle.

———Why I wrote this Field Manual———

This book is the field manual I wish I had as I struggled through the aftermath of service and combat. As soldiers, we undergo one of humanity's most profound cultural initiations. Yet, where warrior-soldiers throughout history were carefully reintegrated into their communities after service, today's veterans sign discharge papers and are cast adrift into a world barely aware of its own military. We are either lionized or pathologized, but rarely understood as members reemerging from a fundamentally different culture.

The wounds we carry—physical, psychological, neurological, and spiritual—run deeper than most civilians can see. We face the alienation of losing the tightest bonds we'll likely ever know, the lingering consequences of injuries and repeated blast and chemical exposures, and a constellation of symptoms more complex than the "shell-shocked veteran" stereotype. Sadly, sometimes the trauma comes from within the ranks through sexual assault, physical assault, bullying, harassment, or discrimination.

Since 9/11, veteran suicides have outnumbered combat deaths, with veterans dying by suicide at nearly twice the civilian rate, yet most never had a PTSD diagnosis, revealing how incomplete our current understanding of the veteran experience is. This continues a tragic pattern across generations: the original dismissal of PTSD, Agent Orange, burn pit exposure, etc. Time and again, veterans have had to fight for recognition of the injuries sustained in service.

Today, more than 500,000 veterans of the Global War on Terror have been diagnosed with PTSD, and thousands are forced to travel abroad for life-saving psychedelic treatments unavailable at home due to outdated laws. We face our most devastating crisis yet.

I founded Heroic Hearts Project and wrote this manual because psychedelics saved my life when conventional treatments failed. Like so many veterans, I had tried everything to escape the spiral into darkness. We're always clear that psychedelics aren't for everyone, but conventional mental health care is failing too many of us. The need for an urgent and radical response could not be greater.

This manual reminds veterans that our struggles aren't personal failings, but the natural fallout of military conditioning meeting civilian life. It is written for veterans seeking a way forward, for families trying to understand why their loved one seems like a stranger, for clinicians searching for better approaches, and for anyone asking why more of us are lost to suicide than to combat. The chapters ahead provide the tactical intelligence to help you understand your mind, evaluate your options, and execute a recovery mission that just might save your life.

CHAPTER 2

SO YOU'RE OUT OF THE MILITARY

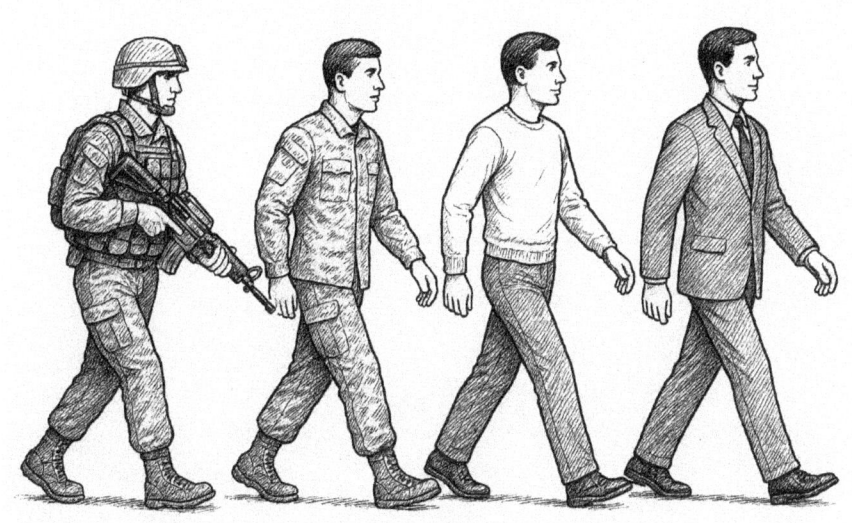

*Life after service can be harder than you thought,
leading to feelings of alienation.*

So you are out of the military. This is not as easy as you thought it would be. And that's not on you. That's a universal experience many of us have gone through.

You came into this very young. You had to mature in specific ways very quickly. You were at the front and center of geopolitical change, bringing you purpose in a way few other jobs can.

You were surrounded by people of the same mindset, who possibly became closer to you than family, thanks to bonds forged in intense training and life-and-death situations.

When you leave, you're unlikely to find the same bonds in corporate, university, or other civilian worlds. You lived with an intensity of experience, purpose, and even transcendence that could be as thrilling as it was terrifying. That can be fun—badass.

But once you get home, life doesn't hit as hard.

Not only that, you are also dealing with possible trauma from your service, whether it be PTSD, moral injury, grief from the death of loved ones, loss of community and purpose, or physical, psychological, or brain injury.

It's challenging to engage with the people around you who see the military as a "necessary evil," or something to put in the past and shut up about. But you're forever changed after service; how do you pretend it never happened?

Welcome to the transition. This is much harder than you thought it would be. Psychedelic-assisted therapy can serve as an important piece of the transition puzzle.

Why Heroic Hearts Project advocates for psychedelic healing for veterans

The day you leave the military, you join America's almost 20 million veterans. For many, this transition marks the beginning of an unexpected battle with the psychological aftermath of service in a mental health system ill-equipped to understand or address the complexity of challenges veterans face.

The reality for post-9/11 veterans is bleak. Four times as many have died from suicide as in combat, with between 17 and 44 estimated to be dying by their own hand each day. Although veterans represent less than 10 percent of the U.S. population, they account for nearly a quarter of its suicides. Suicide rates among those who served have increased by *60–65 percent* since the Global War on Terrorism began. Additionally, their rates of addiction and mental health issues are at record-high levels.

Why veterans need psychedelic and MDMA therapies

- Four times as many veterans have died from suicide as in combat (Suitt, 2021).
- It is estimated that between 17 and 44 veterans die by their own hand each day (U.S. Department of Veterans Affairs, 2024; America's Warrior Partnership, 2022).
- Although veterans make up less than 10 percent of the U.S. adult population, they account for roughly 14 percent of all adult suicide deaths (Ruiz et al., 2023).
- Veteran suicide rates have increased by approximately 60-65 percent since the Global War on Terror began in 2001 (U.S. Department of Veterans Affairs, 2024; Kittel et al., 2025).
- Veterans continue to experience addiction and mental health issues at rates significantly higher than their civilian counterparts (Ngo et al., 2025; Moore et al., 2025; Miller, 2025).

If you're a veteran reading this, you've probably lost one or more teammates to suicide. You've seen others spiral into addiction or become estranged from their loved ones. Maybe that veteran is you, and you're hanging on by the skin of your teeth, wondering how you got this way. These are the veterans we bring into psychedelic healing through HHP.

While PTSD is a clinical condition, it is also an oversimplified catch-all for a spectrum of issues we face. In fact, a significant number of those who died by suicide *had no PTSD diagnosis.*

Today's veterans grapple with challenges beyond PTSD that include moral injury, persistent grief, the abrupt loss of community, a sudden loss of purpose and prestige, metabolic breakdown, and chronic symptoms of brain and bodily injury.

Additionally, the discharged service member faces a double exile: the first from an ancient tradition that reshaped their identity and the second from a detached civilian population that either ignores, misunderstands, or criticizes their experiences. Few understand that this chasm between military and civilian cultures is a historical aberration, the concept of "civilian" being a relatively recent social development. The result is that today's veterans, transformed by peak experiences, ancient rites, and deep bonds of service, find themselves adrift in a world of indifference and alienation.

HHP argues that veterans, conditioned through military service to navigate extreme states of consciousness, are already adept at psychedelic healing work. They are well-versed in accessing profound transformative experiences through the intense collective ceremonies of military life. Although military service is now industrialized and corporatized, it nevertheless harkens back to an age-old lineage of ritual, ceremony, and mythology, practices that mirror millennia of psychedelic traditions across cultures. The warrior's path and the shamanic journey share roots in humanity's earliest understanding of transcendent states of being, long before a "civilian society" developed. These rites emerged from our earliest human ancestors, who banded together for hunting, defense, and survival, and who intuitively understood that threshold experiences—whether in defense, ceremony, or the collective hunt—transformed consciousness in ways essential to human survival. Those ancestral roots are still very much alive in our DNA.

In the ceremonial psychedelic healing space, veterans can reconnect with and integrate the warrior archetype not as a wound to be healed but as an inherent aspect of our collective survival. This stands in stark contrast to the West's industrial medical model, which reduces spiritual and existential crises to clinical diagnoses, medicating and pathologizing the veteran's experience. Yes, service can inflict genuine psychological and spiritual injuries, but this does not corrupt the underlying nobility of the *calling* to serve.

─────Why psychedelics work─────

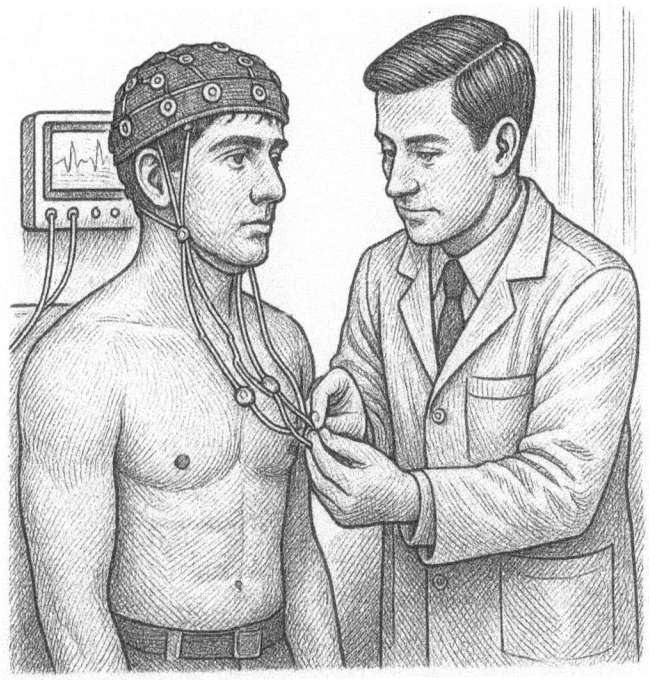

Psychedelic and MDMA therapies interrupt the negative patterns of PTSD and other mental health disorders and allow you to create new, healthier ones. Some psychedelics have also been shown to support healing from brain injury.

PTSD, depression, anxiety, substance abuse, moral injury, alienation, and other mental health issues stemming from service trauma can turn the veteran's psyche into a neurological prison. The individual feels trapped in mental "loops" that become sickeningly more efficient over time. Throw in chronic neurological inflammation from brain trauma, and you have a brain wired for hypervigilance and hypersensitivity while trapped in a downward spiral of despair, depression, and shame. For too many veterans, suicide became the only route to relief.

Researchers suggest the psychedelic mystical experience interrupts these imprisoning mental loops and allows the individual to step outside of their habitual thought patterns. This enables them to process and revisit their thoughts and emotions from a more neutral and accepting vantage point.

Effectiveness of psychedelic and MDMA therapies
1. MDMA-assisted psychotherapy showed a 67% efficacy rate in studies
2. Lasting healing has been seen in one to several sessions
3. No long-term side effects have been identified
4. Shown to help process unresolved trauma versus only masking symptoms
5. Significant improvement to quality of life has been demonstrated in patients
6. Treatment quickly and significantly reduces suicidality
7. Results are rapidly evident

Consider the following regarding psychedelic healing and MDMA-assisted therapy:

1. In a landmark trial, 67 percent of participants receiving MDMA-assisted psychotherapy no longer met diagnostic criteria for PTSD two months after treatment (Mitchell et al., 2021), compared to the 20–30 percent efficacy rates typically seen with antidepressants (Stein et al., 2006).

2. While medications require daily use, sometimes indefinitely, psychedelic-assisted therapy promotes lasting healing in just one to several therapeutic sessions (Carhart-Harris & Goodwin, 2017; Carhart-Harris et al., 2018).

3. Psychedelic therapies do not cause long-term side effects in the way medications like SSRIs, antipsychotics, and mood stabilizers frequently do, such as weight gain, sexual dysfunction, drowsiness, and cognitive dulling. Psychedelic therapies, in contrast, generally do not require long-term dosing and thus reduce the risk of such side effects (Carhart-Harris et al., 2016; Mithoefer et al., 2018).

4. Psychedelic therapies work better by helping veterans process and release unresolved trauma, versus masking or dulling symptoms like medications do (Sessa, 2017).

5. Psychedelic therapies profoundly improve patients' quality of life and allow them to genuinely recover, versus numbing pain. Seventy-four percent of veterans who received MDMA-assisted therapy reported maintaining significant improvements in PTSD symptoms and overall well-being (Mithoefer et al., 2013; Ot'alora et al., 2018).

6. Even a single psilocybin session, combined with psychotherapy, has been

shown to produce rapid and sustained reductions in depression and anxiety, outcomes strongly associated with reduced suicidality (Griffiths et al., 2016).

7. Psychedelic therapies work rapidly to improve mood and relieve symptoms compared to medications that can take weeks or even months to become effective. This is life-changing for veterans at the end of their rope (Carhart-Harris et al., 2018).

While psychedelics are not for everyone, we advocate for their legitimacy and legalization for the veteran community because we have seen and experienced their efficacy dramatically surpass that of conventional treatments like medications.

———Stepping onto a new path———

A frequent refrain we hear is that psychedelics kick the door open, but you must walk through it. The psychedelic- and MDMA-assisted therapy models are not a "one and done" or "take a pill for a symptom" approach. Instead, they are catalysts for a new path that includes community, integration, and continuous personal growth. They also foster an appreciation of the inner "warrior archetype" that drew many to military service in the first place.

This path requires evolving beyond the narrow rules of the conventional medical paradigm into which we've all been indoctrinated. While modern medicine is miraculous in acute situations, medication often masks symptoms instead of providing lasting healing.

For example, if the "check engine" light comes on in your car, you don't put duct tape over the light. Instead, you pop the hood and figure out the problem to avoid engine failure.

The psychedelic therapy approach is similar. We must recognize symptoms as warning signs of deeper issues and tackle the root causes instead of masking them with medications, alcohol, drugs, or self-sabotage. HHP is not anti-medicine; we're pro-sustainable healing. It might seem overwhelming when you're just trying to get through each day, but once that door is opened, most people can't wait to walk through it and find their purpose again. The beauty of this system is that when veterans begin their healing journey, they often feel compelled to take on service roles within the community or reach out to others they know who are suffering and introduce them to this path.

Veterans must advocate
for recognition and care

HHP's efforts to help veterans in crisis are the latest in a long line of grassroots initiatives to provide basic care for our veterans, who have made profound sacrifices on behalf of civilians.

For generations, U.S. veterans have shouldered the costs of our nation's wars, only to return home and face a new, often unseen battle in navigating the maze of inadequate care. What began with early PTSD support groups has evolved into an ongoing struggle for access to modern, life-saving therapies, including psychedelic treatments. Veterans continue to carry the burden of advocating for the recognition and care they need for recovery.

Basic care and recognition that veterans have had to fight for over the years
• Trauma and PTSD • Agent Orange exposure consequences • Burn pit exposure consequences • The post-9/11 suicide crisis

The history of veterans' health advocacy is a tale of neglect and perseverance. In the early years of the Vietnam War, veterans displaying signs of psychological trauma were dismissed by VA psychiatrists and their claims were denied. Desperate for support, veterans formed mutual aid groups. It wasn't until 1980, through the efforts of veteran advocates, psychiatrists, and new research, that PTSD was officially recognized as a diagnosable condition in the Diagnostic and Statistical Manual of Mental Disorders (DSM-III).

Vietnam veterans faced another crisis in the form of Agent Orange, which was linked to multiple mysterious and life-threatening symptoms. It took decades of veteran advocacy before the government finally acknowledged the connection and provided the necessary care. By then, many had already succumbed to disease, and even today, some veteran groups are still fighting for recognition and compensation related to Agent Orange exposure.

This pattern repeated itself when the government dismissed the link between burn pit exposure and the health problems reported by Iraq and Afghanistan veterans. Once again, it took years of advocacy, veteran-led marches to

Congress, and high-profile campaigns to document the devastating effects, organize, and demand recognition and care from policymakers.

Currently, our veterans face the worst crisis yet. Since September 11, 2001, approximately 150,000 veterans have died by suicide, a number that should haunt every one of us. For every U.S. service member killed in combat since then, **about four veterans have died by suicide** (Suitt, 2021). This is the clearest, most damning sign of our failure to provide veterans with proper mental health care.

Traditional treatments are simply not working for many, and the system's response has been slow, bureaucratic, and inadequate.

The good news is that psychedelic and MDMA-assisted therapies have shown tremendous promise in treating PTSD. Yet here we are, once again battling entrenched bureaucratic barriers to fight for recognition and access to therapies that work. While we selflessly sacrificed our physical and mental health to serve our country, our country conveniently discards us when it's done with us.

However, a new generation is stepping up to demand a future where our struggles are acknowledged, our needs prioritized, and our voices heard. *This book aims to illuminate that path, exploring how psychedelic healing offers a chance to reclaim dignity, purpose, and connection.*

It's time we honor the sacrifices of those who have served, not just in words, but in meaningful action.

"People always say thank you for your service, but I'm fed up with my friends and former teammates dying by suicide," said one Army Ranger veteran. "If you want to thank us, give us access to a therapy that is actually saving lives."

CHAPTER 3

TWELVE THINGS CIVILIANS GET WRONG ABOUT VETERANS

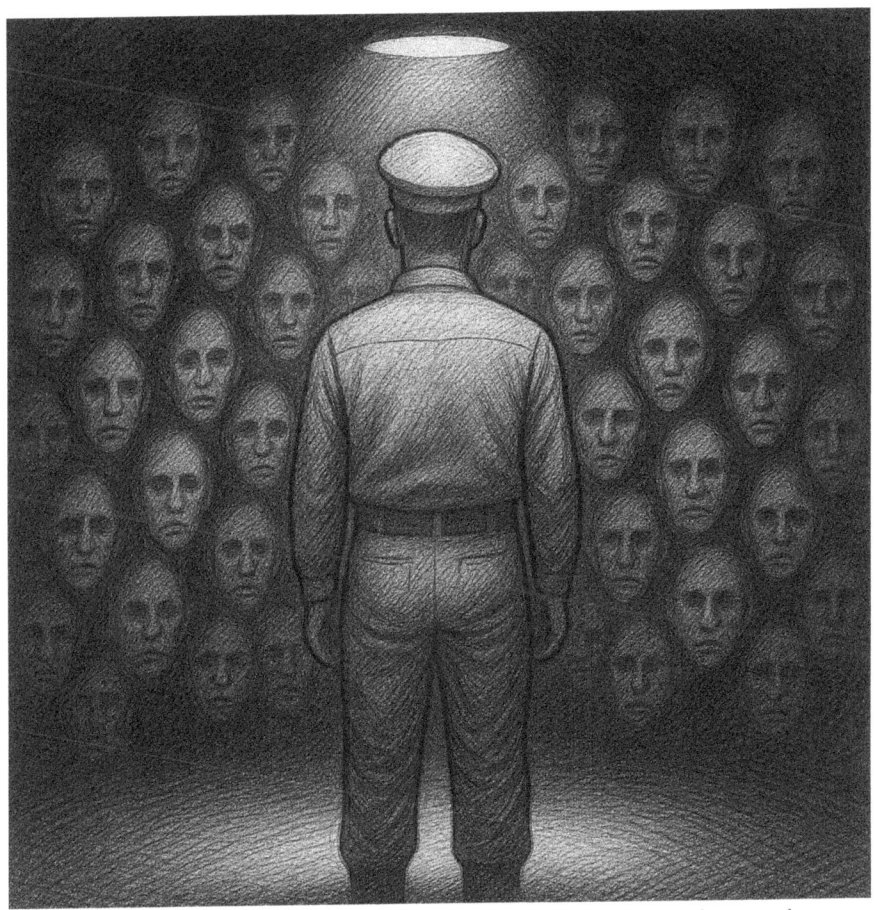

The disconnect between military and civilian cultures is historically unique, with civilians frequently misunderstanding the military experience.

For civilians reading this book, understanding common misconceptions can help you better support the veterans in your life. Many well-meaning civilians have assumptions that miss the mark and can complicate the healing process.

Twelve things civilians get wrong about veterans

1. You can only get PTSD in combat
2. Saying, "Thank you for your service," covers your responsibility
3. Telling veterans to just get over it
4. All veterans are broken
5. Military culture is a temporary identity
6. All veterans are the same
7. Veteran mental health is just about trauma
8. Military service is just a job
9. Veterans want to forget
10. Healing means becoming a civilian
11. Veterans don't belong in psychedelic spaces or deserve psychedelic healing
12. Psychedelics will make veterans "soft"

————Key misunderstandings to be aware of————

1. Combat and PTSD
Not every veteran has PTSD, and not every veteran with service-related trauma was in combat. While combat trauma is significant, many veterans struggle with moral injury, grief, identity loss, and other challenges unrelated to direct combat exposure. Additionally, many veterans with PTSD developed it from non-combat traumas like military sexual assault or training accidents.

2. "Thank you for your service"
While well-intentioned, this phrase makes some veterans struggling with moral injury or complex feelings about their service uncomfortable.

3. "Just get over it"
The military experience fundamentally transforms identity and worldview in ways that can't simply be left behind. Telling veterans to "move on" or "get over it" dismisses the profound nature of this transformation.

4. The broken veteran narrative
Media portrayals often present veterans as either damaged victims or unstable threats. This binary thinking misses the complex reality of the post-military service experience and can make veterans feel alienated or misunder-

stood. Many veterans are neither broken nor dangerous. Instead, they're navigating a complex cultural transition while processing experiences civilians can't relate to.

5. Military culture is temporary
Many civilians view military service as something veterans need to leave behind to reintegrate into civilian life. Military service can create a permanent and profound transformation. Veterans don't need to abandon their military identity to heal. Instead, they need to find ways to integrate it meaningfully into their civilian life.

6. All veterans are the same
Veterans are not a monolith. Their experiences, beliefs, and needs are as diverse as their branch of service, era of service, role, deployments, and countless other factors.

7. Veteran mental health is just about trauma
While trauma plays a role in veteran mental health, many veterans struggle more with loss of purpose, community disconnection, or difficulty translating their skills to civilian life. Focusing solely on trauma overlooks these challenges.

8. Military service is just a job
Civilians often equate leaving military service with changing careers or moving to a new apartment. This overlooks how military service reshapes one's identity, worldview, and sense of purpose. The military isn't just what veterans did, it becomes part of who they are.

9. Veterans want to forget
Many civilians assume veterans want to forget or avoid talking about their service. While some might, many veterans would appreciate having their service understood and integrated into their life story, rather than being hidden away or ignored.

10. Healing means becoming a civilian
True healing for veterans doesn't mean becoming "more civilian." It means integrating their military identity with civilian life. The goal isn't to erase the warrior but to help them find their place in peace.

11. Veterans don't belong in psychedelic spaces or deserve psychedelic healing
Psychedelics have been shown to be very effective in treating the traumas unique to veterans' experiences. Their military background of ceremony,

ritual, discipline, and peak experiences makes veterans ideal candidates for psychedelic therapeutic approaches. Veterans are not a monolith; every person enlists for different reasons. It's detrimental to use political leanings and belief systems to deny anyone access to healing.

12. Psychedelics will make veterans soft

Others worry that psychedelic experiences will make veterans "soft" or compromise their warrior spirit. Psychedelics don't erase the warrior, but rather, they help veterans integrate their warrior identity. Many report emerging with greater wisdom about when and how to apply their warrior training.

————Conclusion————

Understanding these misconceptions shapes how we approach veteran healing. When we recognize that military service creates a permanent cultural transformation rather than temporary trauma, we can better support veterans in integrating their experiences rather than trying to "fix" them. This understanding is integral to psychedelic healing work, where honoring rather than pathologizing the military experience creates space for transformation.

CHAPTER 4

WHY YOU'RE SUFFERING:
THE PTSD-ISH UMBRELLA

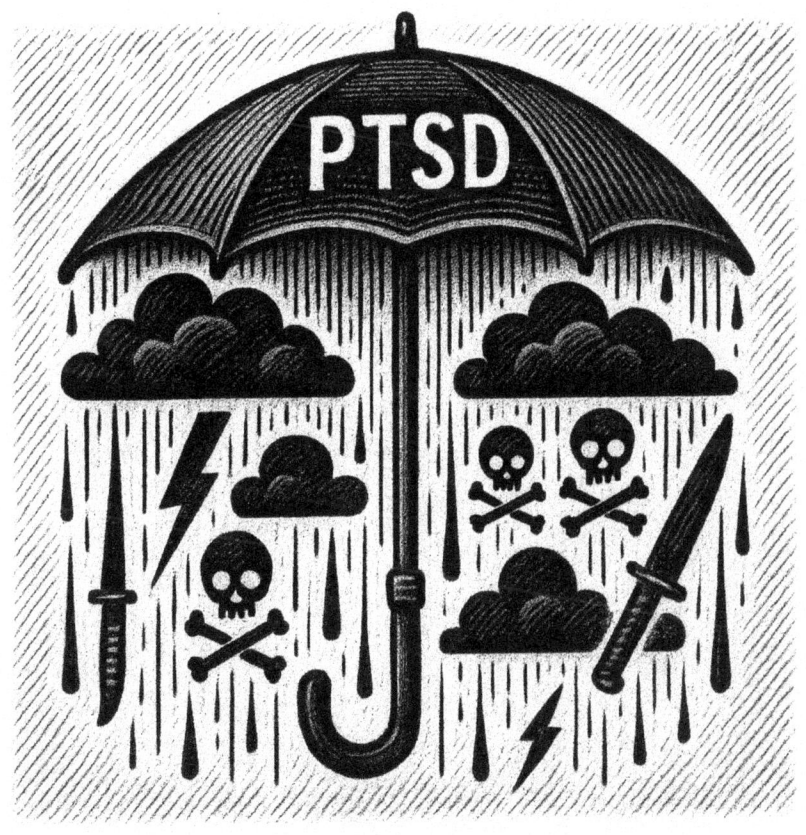

PTSD is often used as an umbrella term for the multiple mental health issues veterans face. In fact, most veterans who died by suicide did not have a PTSD diagnosis.

PTSD only explains one part of what causes veterans to suffer. At HHP, we use the term PTSD so the public can understand our mission. In truth, we're also focused on lesser-known factors such as moral injury, grief, shame, loss of community, alienation, and metabolic, physical, and neurological injuries.

———The "promise" of psychedelic healing———

There is controversy over how to present the psychedelic-healing paradigm to the public. Some researchers worry advocates are overly enthusiastic, oversell the promises, and downplay the risks.

However, HHP operates with a sense of *urgency.* More than forty veterans take their lives each day in the U.S. (rates are high in other countries as well). While we, too, shun glamorizing psychedelics or making empty promises, our community does not have the luxury of being overly cautious.

Additionally, we are combating sixty years of untruthful and damaging propaganda about psychedelics. However, when you experience or witness psychedelic healing firsthand, it's unlike anything in the pharmaceutical model. This makes people naturally enthusiastic, but we consistently emphasize realistic expectations and the need for patients to put in their own work.

In this chapter, we'll go over some of the common factors that contribute to suicide and other mental health issues, and why psychedelic therapy is uniquely beneficial in addressing them.

————Post-traumatic stress disorder (PTSD)————

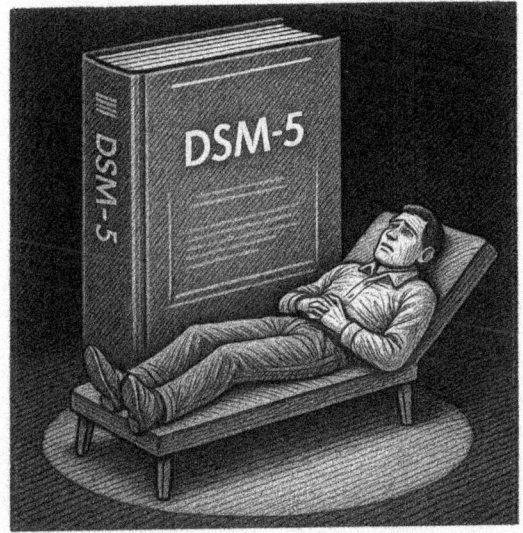

Many factors other than combat can cause PTSD in veterans. PTSD affects up to an estimated 30 percent of post-9/11 veterans compared to about 6 percent of civilians.

While combat exposure is the most recognizable cause of veteran PTSD, it can also come through military sexual trauma, witnessing or experiencing training accidents, being bullied by fellow team members, or exposure to death and human remains during humanitarian missions. PTSD affects up to almost 30 percent of post-9/11 veterans compared to about 6 percent of civilians (U.S. Department of Veterans Affairs, 2025).

Common causes of PTSD among veterans
• Combat
• Non-combat service roles
• Injuries, deaths, or other traumas during training
• Head injuries
• Military sexual trauma
• Exclusion, bullying, harassment, or assault from fellow team members during service
• Trauma during humanitarian missions

The VA initially screens for PTSD with the Primary Care PTSD Screen (PC-PTSD-5). If the indications are positive, veterans are given a more comprehensive screening that aligns with diagnostic criteria. Other conditions, such as traumatic brain injury (TBI), depression, and substance use disorders, are also evaluated since they frequently co-occur with PTSD.

Primary Care PTSD Screen (PC-PTSD-5)
Have you experienced any of the following in the past month?

- Had nightmares about the event(s) or thought about the event(s) when you did not want to?
- Tried hard not to think about the event(s) or went out of your way to avoid situations that reminded you of the event(s)?
- Been constantly on guard, watchful, or easily startled?
- Felt numb or detached from people, activities, or your surroundings?
- Felt guilty or unable to stop blaming yourself or others for the event(s) or any problems the event(s) may have caused?

First-line treatments through the VA include trauma-focused therapies, medication management, and complementary approaches such as meditation, outdoor therapy, service dog programs, and peer support groups. While the VA estimates about a 50–60 percent rate of symptom reduction, the dropout rate is also as high as 40 percent. Limited access to care, lack of culturally competent providers, and complex patient cases further hinder success rates. Additionally, only about 50 percent of veterans with PTSD seek treatment through the VA.

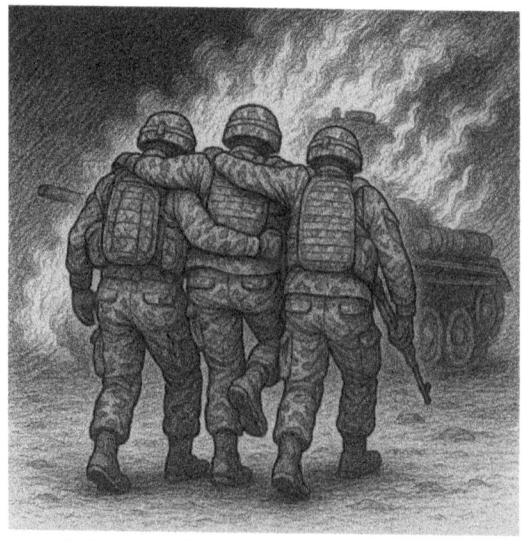

Only about 50 percent of veterans with PTSD seek treatment through the VA.

How psychedelics and MDMA-assisted therapy have helped veterans heal from PTSD

Psychedelics and MDMA appear to reduce activity in the brain's amygdala (fear center) while increasing connectivity between brain regions involved in memory and emotional regulation. This may help veterans process traumatic memories with less emotional overwhelm.

Psychedelics appear to create a window of neural plasticity that allows veterans to:

- Access and process traumatic memories without becoming emotionally triggered or overwhelmed
- Develop new perspectives on their experiences
- Create healthier neural patterns around trauma triggers
- Release stored trauma from the body

Additionally, research thus far has shown that MDMA-assisted therapy results in almost 70 percent of participants no longer meeting PTSD criteria after treatment (Mitchell et al., 2021).

In a therapeutic setting, MDMA:

- Reduces fear while accessing difficult memories
- Increases self-compassion and reduces shame
- Allows access to previously blocked memories
- Helps participants find meaning in their experiences

In December 2024, the Department of Veterans Affairs began enrolling veterans in its first psychedelic-assisted therapy trial in more than fifty years, a $1.5 million, five-year study testing MDMA-assisted psychotherapy for PTSD and alcohol use disorder at VA medical centers in Providence, Rhode Island, and West Haven, Connecticut, in partnership with researchers from Brown and Yale universities.

———Moral Injury———

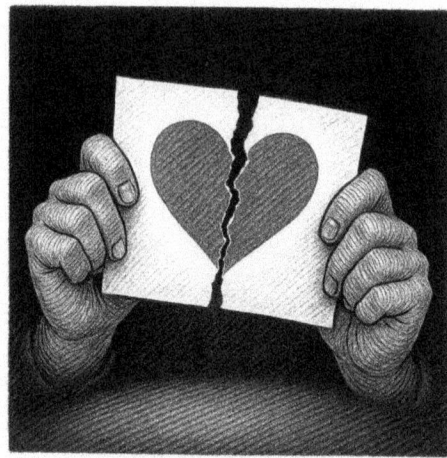

Moral injury, defined as trauma caused by acting against one's beliefs or values, is a common consequence of service and combat.

Moral injury, the trauma caused by acting against one's beliefs or values, may be the most significant, least understood, and most challenging mental health disorder to treat in the current veteran mental health crisis.

Moral injury distinguishes military-related trauma from most other kinds and can result in guilt, shame, depression, anger, and existential crisis, sometimes to a crippling degree. It is not the same as PTSD, although the two can co-exist. Multiple facets of combat and service can contribute to moral injury.

Causes of moral injury in the combat zone

- Inflicting violence
- Witnessing the violent deaths of comrades
- Witnessing or being the cause of civilian suffering
- Having to make critical moral decisions without sufficient preparation or training
- Inability to prevent harm to others
- Confronting complex moral situations (e.g., child combatants)
- Repeated deployments with insufficient recovery time or while injured/brain-injured
- Repeated separation from family

Although there are no standardized diagnostic criteria for moral injury, conventional treatments include:

- Adaptive Disclosure Therapy
- Impact of Killing Treatment
- Modified Cognitive Processing Therapy
- Acceptance and Commitment Therapy

Current treatments have success rates of 35 to 50 percent in reducing symptoms. However, success is difficult to define, as symptoms overlap with other disorders, and moral injury includes spiritual and existential elements that are difficult to measure. As with other forms of conventional treatment, success rates are also hampered by high dropout rates and varying accessibility.

Symptoms of moral injury
While symptoms of moral injury and PTSD can overlap, moral injury focuses on ethical and spiritual responses rather than fear-based trauma responses.

The term "moral injury" was coined by Dr. Jonathan Shay in his 1994 book *Achilles in Vietnam*, in which he compared the psychological wounds of Vietnam veterans to the warriors in Homer's *Iliad*. He illustrated how the moral injury of war has remained consistent throughout human history.

Despite significant advances in treating trauma, the U.S. government's ability to help veterans heal from moral injury lags far behind its capacity to prepare and deploy them for combat.

THE VETERAN'S FIELD MANUAL FOR PSYCHEDELICS

Common symptoms of moral injury include:
• Persistent and profound guilt and shame
• Feelings of betrayal and anger at leadership or institutions
• Loss of trust in authority figures and institutions
• Inability to forgive oneself
• Feelings of being morally irredeemable
• Loss of faith or spiritual crisis
• Questioning the meaning of life and death
• Social withdrawal and isolation
• Self-destructive and self-sabotaging behaviors
• Difficulty forming or maintaining close relationships
• Self-punishment
• Intrusive thoughts about moral violations
• Persistent self-questioning
• Feeling unworthy or "broken"
• Preoccupation with amends or redemption
• Difficulty integrating wartime experiences into one's life narrative

Shame and guilt: The poisons of moral injury

Mental health professionals cite shame and guilt as the two most prominent aspects of moral injury.

Normally, shame alerts individuals to perceived moral or social violations, helping maintain appropriate behavior within human societies. While this response can encourage corrective action, when it occurs too often or too intensely, it may overactivate the amygdala, leading to social anxiety, avoidance, and other mental health problems (Cibich et al., 2016).

"We particularly see this in driven individuals who excel at problem-solving, as these personality types also tend to ruminate and fall into negative thought cycles," said Robert Koffman, MD, MPH, CAPT, MC, USN (RET.). "Shame and guilt are significant components of moral injury and are challenging to treat. Current protocols are ridiculously ineffective."

Betrayal

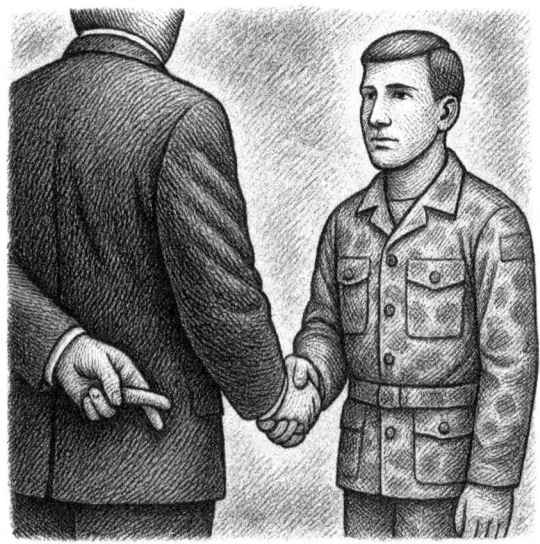

Betrayal plays a significant role in many cases of moral injury and can stem from many sources.

Betrayal plays a significant role in many cases of moral injury and can stem from many sources. Below are some of the more common causes of betrayal that lead to moral injury in veterans.

Institutional betrayal

Many enlisted during the Iraq and Afghanistan wars with noble intentions to defend and protect the United States, and recruits are rigorously indoctrinated into high moral values and codes like honor, loyalty, and integrity during boot camp.

Over time, a significant number felt that their ideals and values had been exploited. The Iraq War was launched based on false evidence, military decisions were made by politicians with no war experience, and lower-ranking soldiers involved in the Abu Ghraib scandal were punished while senior officers were protected. Additionally, soldiers were deployed believing they were serving a humanitarian mission to protect civilians and help rebuild communities, a contrast to the actual role of seeking out and killing the enemy.

Twenty years of seemingly endless warfare and multiple false promises left many veterans feeling used and betrayed. This came to a crescendo with the fall of Kabul, Afghanistan, in 2021. Thousands of soldiers endured years of sacrifice and grievous injury, watched friends die, and witnessed or participated in the deaths of innocent civilians, only to have the country handed back to the Taliban overnight.

Additionally, they were forced to leave behind interpreters, cultural advisors, and other Afghan allies—many of whom had become close friends—to be tortured and executed by the Taliban after years of being promised protection. This created profound moral wounds for many veterans.

After the fall of Kabul, many veterans reported intense feelings of betrayal, guilt, humiliation, and anger over the war's outcome and concern for Afghan allies. Some VA sources and surveys indicate an increase in veterans seeking mental health support in response to these emotions.

Unfortunately, betrayal by the politicians in command is something militaries have grappled with throughout history.

Julius Caesar launched campaigns more for personal power than necessity, while the farms of his deployed soldiers fell into debt and were seized by politicians, leaving them impoverished upon their return.

Napoleon abandoned his army in Russia, leaving hundreds of thousands to die while he rushed back to Paris to protect his political position.

After the Civil War, Union veterans had to fight for years to receive their pensions, while Confederate veterans were left largely destitute. Many ended up in poor houses.

After World War I, American veterans were denied promised bonuses during the Great Depression, leading to the tragic Bonus Army march, where troops were ordered to attack their fellow veterans.

President Bush sent U.S. forces into Afghanistan with a story to democratize Afghanistan, but he never had an exit strategy. Both Presidents Obama and Trump promised to get U.S. troops out of Afghanistan, but neither did because it would have been a political catastrophe. Indeed, it was a catastrophe when the U.S. finally pulled out under President Biden.

The disconnect between politicians and the military results in politicians rarely facing the human costs of their decisions.

Tactical betrayal
Many U.S. veterans had cultivated relationships with Afghan allies who were later left behind to suffer retaliation from the Taliban.

At the same time, troops were betrayed by Afghan allies or civilians, some of them children, who gained their trust only to place IEDs or feed strategic information to insurgents. In some cases, soldiers were forced to fire on armed child combatants who threatened the lives of their entire team, leading to a lasting fear of children long after their service ended.

Troops trained and served with Afghan soldiers who kept young boys to abuse sexually (*bacha bazi*, a prevalent practice in Afghanistan).

These situations forced soldiers into impossible choices for which they were not prepared and that violated their values, haunting them for years afterward.

Leadership and logistical betrayal

Troops were sent to war in Iraq and Afghanistan with insufficient manpower, resources, and equipment to withstand battle. It took grassroots efforts spearheaded by troops' family members and supporters to provoke a government response. Due to the length of the war and lack of manpower, soldiers went through multiple rapid deployments despite injuries, TBIs, or severe psychological distress.

Military codes of honor and loyalty shielded a leadership deeply corroded by decades of war. Studies showed that the leadership culture had become "ethically numb," thrusting troops into split-second moral decisions for which they were not trained or prepared (Wong & Gerras, 2015).

Public betrayal

Moral injury from war is a collective wound, yet a historically unprecedented divide has emerged between civilian and military life. While troops in Iraq and Afghanistan fought and died through twenty years of war, the public drifted into complacent detachment. Never before has a nation been so insulated from the moral weight of its wars while a small volunteer force carried the full burden.

This societal disconnect forces veterans to grapple alone with moral injury while surrounded by a society that, at best, doesn't understand or share the consequences of war and, at worst, chastises veterans. As Sebastian Junger observes in his book *Tribe*, soldiers often return to find that, "although they're willing to die for their country, they're not sure how to live for it" (Junger, 2016). This disconnect is made more painful by what Junger describes as a society "basically at war with itself," where citizens view each other with contempt rather than the unity that characterized tribal societies of the past.

Squad betrayal

For veterans who are women, people of color, and LGBTQ+, the betrayal came from within their units. Bullying, assault, harassment, discrimination, violence, and exclusion meant some soldiers were fighting both on the field and in the barracks. Those who reported assault or harassment, often at the hands of their superiors, frequently faced various forms of retaliation. As a result, the rates of PTSD, moral injury, and other mental health disorders are significantly higher in these populations.

Killing

Moral injury frequently stems from the act of killing, witnessing, or causing the deaths of civilians and team members. Many struggle with survivor's guilt from having come home alive when teammates didn't. Even witnessing or causing the death of animals in the war zones haunts many veterans.

Death is inherent to the job of war, and it's important to note this doesn't affect all equally. Some combat soldiers view killing as a regular part of their duties and feel either neutral or even positive about it. Others may have mixed feelings, but their training desensitized and conditioned them for such actions. Others are persistently haunted by it.

Moral injury frequently stems from the act of causing or witnessing death.

Research shows that killing in combat is a significant predictor of PTSD symptoms, alcohol abuse, anger, relationship problems, and higher rates of suicidal ideation than that of veterans with no combat killing experiences (Kelley et al., 2019; Tokar, 2010).

The neurology of killing

Our response to threats is a primitive, involuntary mechanism developed over millennia. The brain protects soldiers during combat by releasing self-protective neurochemicals such as adrenaline, dopamine, and endorphins. These feel-good chemicals can induce a rewarding, euphoric, and zen-like state of flow. A life-and-death setting also bonds soldiers in ways few other life experiences will.

Combined, these scenarios can put a positive spin on combat. However, once back in the monotony of civilian peacetime, this neurochemical flow state wanes. Unprocessed memories and traumas can settle into the recesses of the psyche, keeping the nervous system on high alert while giving rise to shame, guilt, self-loathing, and depression.

In both the military and civilian worlds, "killing" is often shrouded in euphemisms or sanitized language to distance us from reality. Veterans who killed in combat instinctively avoid discussing the topic with civilians as if to protect them from the "contamination" of killing in war. It's not something one can understand unless they've been through it. This divide makes some veterans feel alienated and misunderstood.

While combat actions make sense in war, they can conflict with one's post-combat civilian identity and values. This dissonance between the warrior and civilian self can cause distress.

Moral injury among non-combat veterans
Most people assume veteran PTSD stems from combat, but the truth is more complex. PTSD, moral injury, and suicidal ideation also impact non-combat veterans. Mental health experts and veterans suggest various reasons for this.

Moral injury among non-combat veterans
• Lack of purpose and loss of identity
• Feelings of powerlessness
• Remote exposure to the brutalities of war
• Perceived stigma
• Unmet expectations
• Loss of community
• Physical injury and TBIs
• Forced into a role for which you're not prepared

Lack of purpose and loss of identity: The military offers a strong sense of identity and purpose. However, non-combat vets may feel their service was less meaningful or impactful. Or they may feel moral injury or survivor's guilt around not having been able to protect those harmed or killed in action.

Feelings of powerlessness: The immediate focus on group survival provides a sense of purpose for combat vets, which may help mitigate the impact of moral injury. In contrast, those in support roles sometimes struggle with feelings of powerlessness or helplessness around the inability to influence life-or-death situations directly. This lack of agency can make the experience more psychologically distressing and difficult to come to terms with.

Remote exposure to the brutalities of war: Drone operators in remote locations, while safe from combat, nevertheless witnessed war's brutality in real-time through their screens. Their operations also resulted in death and injury to both the enemy and civilians. Although this alone can cause profound psychological trauma, it is compounded by feelings of isolation and a lack of camaraderie that can help soldiers cope with war trauma. Many also reported they felt their distress was less legitimate because they weren't in physical danger (Saini et al., 2021; Chappelle et al., 2023).

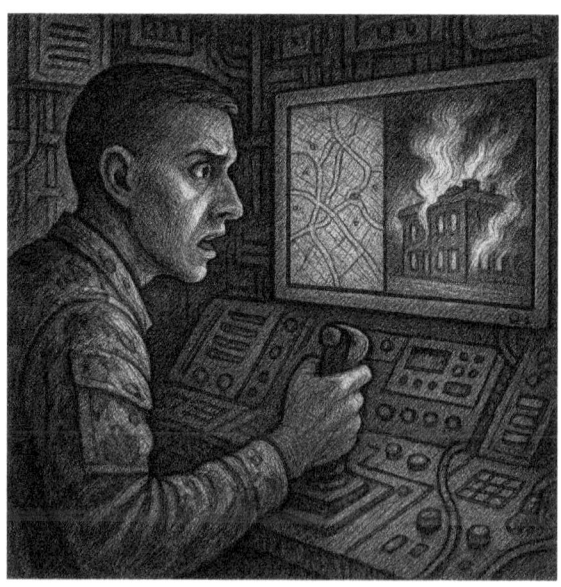

Despite their remote locations, drone operators often suffer from profound psychological trauma.

Unmet expectations: Some veterans enlist because they feel destined for battle. When those expectations go unmet, they often feel deflated or lacking in value upon returning to civilian life.

Loss of community: Most military members form tight bonds and experience a sense of community in service; the high-stress of combat environments often creates an even more lasting bond. Non-combat veterans may have weaker social support systems when they return to civilian life.

Physical injury and TBIs: In 2017, nearly four times as many service members died in training accidents as were killed in combat (Audacy, 2018). Most bodily injuries and TBIs acquired during service happen outside of combat during training exercises, accidents, and routine military activities (U.S. Centers for Disease Control and Prevention [CDC], 2015). These often result from high-risk training activities such as airborne operations, obstacle courses, or live-fire exercises. A significant number of these injuries lead to chronic pain or long-term functional impairment. Injuries sustained during training prevented many soldiers from deploying, contributing to the phenomenon of moral injury.

Perceived stigma: Civilians assume military-related PTSD or other mental health struggles only pertain to combat veterans. The non-combat veteran may feel their mental health struggles are not justified despite the stress, trauma, and increased risk of TBIs and injury in all types of service. As such, they bottle things up and may not seek help.

Forced into a role for which you're not prepared: During the Iraq and Afghanistan wars, many service members were put in roles for which they were not trained. For example, the Navy and Air Force sent augmentees to serve with Army units, where they were often ostracized and isolated, and their rank was disregarded. Service members were assigned to detainee guard forces without receiving proper training to manage detainee violence, hunger strikes, resistance, or self-harm. Military stigma also views the detainee guard service as less honorable. According to some veteran mental health professionals, these individuals often emerge from service with a more pervasive and damaging form of PTSD and moral injury compared to those who served in combat.

Moral injury is not confined to the military

While moral injury is highly prevalent in the military, it is also present in other high-stakes professions, including healthcare, teaching, finance, law enforcement, and social work. Yet, despite being extremely prevalent, it does not appear in the *Diagnostic and Statistical Manual of Mental Disorders (DSM),* which is used to diagnose and dictate insurance coverage. This is another reason it continues to present challenges in awareness and treatment.

Lack of preparation or cleansing to process the psychological impact of killing

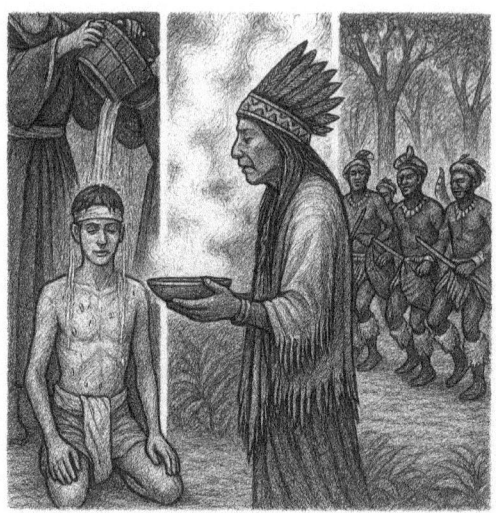

Modern militaries are historically unique in that they do not offer cleansing and purification rituals after combat.

While recruits go through rigorous training to learn how to kill and become desensitized to killing, they are not taught how to process the aftermath, leaving the veteran to process experiences in a vacuum (Kilner, Military Review, 1999). Instead, they are diagnosed with a disorder and medicated, or they seek self-medication through substance abuse or self-destructive habits.

Militaries throughout history recognized the personal dilemmas of warfare and instituted various "cleanses" for returning soldiers. *Miasma*, the spiritual and moral contamination that came from killing or exposure to death, was a common theme in Greek tragedies, requiring ritual purification. Samurai warriors underwent Shinto purification rites, which involved ceremonial washing, specific prayers, offerings at shrines, and ritual gestures. Ancient Hebrews distinguished between combat killing and murder in their laws, and medieval Christian churches required returning soldiers to serve penance. Native American tribes required their returning warriors to go through community-based purification rituals before reentering society. These external processes for killing can help alleviate a soldier's burden and make invisible wounds visible for healing.

The urgent need for community-based psychedelic therapy to address moral injury

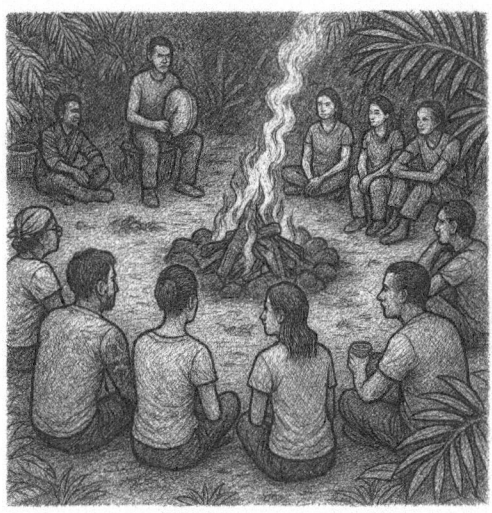

Sacred settings and collective witnessing of the experience can open the door to psychological and spiritual cleansing.

Veteran-only psychedelic and MDMA-assisted group therapy draws on humanity's oldest traditions of providing space for warriors to recover from the psychological and spiritual weight of battle and service. Sacred settings and collective witnessing of the experience can open the door to psychological and spiritual cleansing, honoring the ancient need for soldiers to heal from the unseen wounds of combat.

When veterans are able to prepare, journey, and integrate alongside a community of their peers, psychedelics and MDMA have shown remarkable success in helping them address moral injury.

The journey enables them to process tormenting and traumatic experiences from a place of compassion and self-acceptance. While perpetual shame increasingly distorts trauma in the mind over time, psychedelic therapy allows one to see past events more clearly and free of judgment.

This doesn't mean you will forget these experiences or their gravity; instead, you will get "unstuck" and integrate them without dysregulating the nervous system.

MDMA-assisted therapy, in particular, dampens the activity of the amygdala, the brain's fear center, so memories and traumas can be processed without triggering the fight-or-flight response.

With either MDMA- or psychedelic-assisted therapies, rigid neural networks temporarily dissipate, discharging stored traumas and producing a state of neurological neutrality. From there, the veteran can step off the slow path of self-destruction and begin building a healthier one.

Equally essential is the veteran community itself. Traveling this road with peers with similar struggles can be a profound tool in helping pull you out of the black hole of shame. When you discuss that order to "light up" a white Toyota that was found to carry an innocent family, seeing your best friend's blood soak your uniform, or feeling powerless inside a mission you find unethical, you don't have to worry about censoring yourself like you might with civilians or even non-veteran therapists.

"Veterans have a significant vulnerability when stepping into any kind of caretaking space that isn't of their own culture," said Zach Skiles, PhD, a Marine Corps veteran, psychologist, and psychedelic research coordinator. "You end up with folks who don't understand these nuances, which can complicate a veteran's healing pretty significantly."

———Grief———

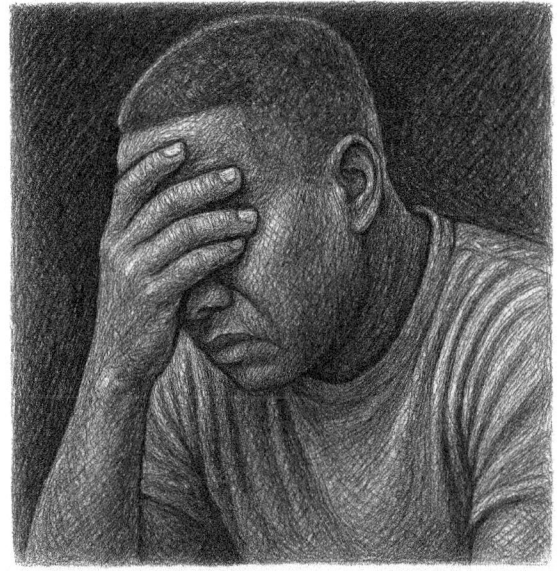

Grief is a normal and healthy response to loss. However, when it becomes Prolonged Grief Disorder, it can threaten your safety or life.

Grief is a common consequence of service. When it impairs daily functioning for more than a year, clinicians may diagnose it as Prolonged Grief Disorder (PGD). The majority of those deployed experienced the deaths of their team members. Non-deployed members also lost teammates to training accidents.

And, of course, we all now face the ongoing loss of our fellow team members to the veteran suicide epidemic.

While all people experience loss and grief, combat grief requires unique understandings and approaches.

Persistent grief disorder may arise from:
• Losing multiple team members simultaneously in combat
• The sudden, violent, or traumatic deaths of teammates
• The inability to prevent combat deaths
• Being unable to recover the body of a fallen teammate
• The need to suppress immediate grief in combat
• The military's culture of stoicism
• Delayed or unavailable grief ritual
• Survivor's guilt
• Feeling civilians don't understand your loss
• Moral injury
• Difficulty integrating combat deaths

Grief is a normal and healthy response to loss. However, it becomes problematic when it threatens your safety or life. Symptoms of PGD include:

- Impaired daily functioning
- Feeling stuck in the grieving process
- Intense longing for fallen comrades that doesn't diminish
- Difficulty accepting the death(s)
- Feeling that part of yourself died, too
- Avoidance of reminders
- Difficulty trusting or connecting with others
- Feeling that life is meaningless without the deceased
- Difficulty engaging in life or planning for the future
- Feeling shame or guilt for not having been able to prevent deaths

Grief within the relationship bonds of service
The pain of service-related grief can feel isolating in a civilian culture that will likely never experience or understand the bonds that develop in war or service. Recruits are indoctrinated to feel responsible for their teammates' lives. The shared hardship and intimacy of communal service strip people to the barest, more raw versions of themselves, often creating deeper bonds than those with spouses or longtime friends. Researchers found that among Vietnam veterans who had lost buddies to combat, the grief of those losses 30 years prior was sometimes more painful than the more recent loss of a spouse (U.S. Department of Veterans Affairs, Grief Recovery Method, 2013).

Additionally, veterans experience "disenfranchised grief" within a civilian society that does not understand or acknowledge their losses, exacerbating the grieving process (Aloi, 2011).

Grief and moral injury

Service-related grief is frequently entangled with questions of meaning, morality, and responsibility. The loss of devoted comrades may be entangled with a sense of betrayal and feeling the loss was meaningless or squandered under false pretenses, which throws the veteran into existential distress over their own purpose. When poor planning, questionable strategies, and inadequate equipment lead to death, it can be challenging to move on from the grip of injustice.

Survivors often carry crushing guilt for having lived or are haunted by questions of whether they could have prevented death in a split-second combat decision. They become trapped in cycles of self-blame or feel they don't deserve to move forward with their lives when their friends who passed didn't get that chance.

Psychedelics and grief

Psychedelic experiences can create profound opportunities for veterans to process grief. In ceremonial spaces, veterans report connecting with lost comrades, confronting survivor's guilt, and finding meaning in their losses. Psychedelic journeys can help veterans break through frozen grief, allowing them to cry openly, release guilt, and discover healthier ways to honor their fallen comrades.

Many veterans have reported that their lost loved ones came to them during psychedelic ceremonies to reassure them that they were okay and to express their wish for their still-living friends to move on and thrive. This can bring enormous relief and peace, helping veterans overcome their grief and guilt.

————Shame————

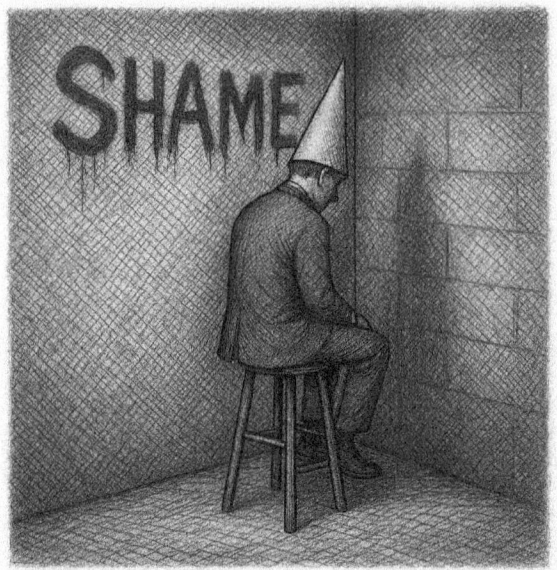

Shame is a common and destructive symptom of PTSD, moral injury, and other service-related mental health disorders.

As introduced earlier, one of the more caustic outcomes of moral injury and PTSD is shame. Shame robs us of the belief that we deserve positive life experiences and disconnects us from loved ones. Furtively working in the recesses of the psyche, it is often expressed as anger, rage, and depression.

Sometimes, it's easy to identify the source of shame. Survivor's guilt is a common cause for veterans. This can be brought on by feeling guilty about not preventing the death or injury of a comrade, or survivors may believe they should have suffered or died instead. For example, a soldier might not have deployed because they were sick or injured, and the person sent in their place was harmed or killed in combat. Support crew members who, while not directly involved in combat, witness traumatic events from command stations. The inability to act in those moments can create a sense of helplessness, magnifying guilt and shame.

A military culture that values stoicism and composure can perpetuate feelings of shame long after discharge. People feel "weak" for not bearing up under the consequences of trauma. For those still serving, admitting to mental health difficulties can jeopardize promotions. Soldiers may feel shame around the fear that they can't live up to the expectations of their fellow soldiers.

In the military, service members often reach peak physical condition while filling roles of clear purpose and responsibility. However, in civilian life, the sudden anonymity can sap self-esteem and foster feelings of shame. Historically, belonging to a soldier or warrior class was highly respected as a lifelong vocation in many cultures, even when individuals were tending to the fields or forging steel in peacetime. Today, however, veterans are abruptly and unceremoniously thrown back into civilian life to navigate this identity crisis alone in a civilian culture blind to their service, sacrifice, and skills. This can foster feelings of shame.

Compass of Shame Theory

Psychologist Donald Nathanson developed the "Compass of Shame Theory" in the 1990s to help illustrate four primary responses to shame (Nathanson, 1998):

North: Attack Self

The internalization of shame by criticizing or blaming oneself leads to self-destructive behaviors or low self-esteem.

East: Attack Others

The direction of shame outward by blaming, criticizing, or lashing out at others to deflect attention from one's feelings.

South: Withdraw

The isolation of oneself, avoidance of social situations or interactions, or shutting down emotionally to escape shame.

West: Avoidance Behaviors

Using denial and distracting activities, such as substance use, thrill-seeking, or compulsive behaviors, to avoid confronting shame directly.

Eventually, the veteran, weighed down by shame, guilt, and moral injury, feels trapped in a neurological prison camp.

Why we feel shame

Our brains use shame as emotional "roadside guideposts" to catalog distressing memories, hoping we don't repeat harmful events. However, under the pressure of traumatic events, these roadside guideposts turn into what Paul Conti, MD, author of *Trauma: The Invisible Epidemic*, calls "roadside bombs." The hypervigilant brain begins to exaggerate shame, irritability, and fear in a self-perpetuating downward spiral. Brain injury and chronic pain—frequent souvenirs of service—exacerbate the symptoms (Conti, 2022).

Secrecy, shame's ugly sibling, turns this poison inward under the guise of self-protection. The two become a slow, poisonous leak, draining energy that could otherwise be used for healing and growth. They feed isolation and reinforce the belief that one is irredeemable, unworthy of help, or undeserving of good things.

As the shame spiral continues, an individual may behave more erratically, make increasingly poor choices, and push away their loved ones. Eventually, the shame may move outward, and others may brand the individual as a loser, weak, addict, rage-aholic, promiscuous, etc., perpetuating the spiral.

Shame and self-hatred unconsciously push us into choices, situations, and relationships that confirm our worst beliefs about ourselves. It's as if some hidden part of us wants the world to see exactly how unworthy we feel.

This is the hardest part about change. When you address your own self-destruction, you've already created an infrastructure that reinforces it. Sometimes, healing requires dismantling the structure that keeps the spiral intact, such as toxic relationships, environments, or habits.

Psychedelics and shame
Shame is a universal experience most people grapple with. Because healthy shame serves a purpose, it's not something psychedelics "cure." However, psychedelic-assisted therapy can help rein in the destruction of excessive shame by guiding you through these aspects of your psyche to confront them. This often leads one through a cathartic breakthrough.

CHAPTER 5

INDIVIDUAL INJURY

Veteran mental health challenges often have physiological roots, with symptoms stemming from multiple body systems damaged by the unique hazards of modern warfare and military training.

Today's service members face an unprecedented combination of threats, including repeated blast exposures, chemical exposures, multiple prescription medications, and the strain of a high-performance culture on hormonal, metabolic, and neurological function.

These physical injuries rarely exist in isolation. Instead, they compound and amplify each other, typically escaping detection in the conventional medical model. For instance, a brain injury impairs emotional regulation, promoting substance use, which further damages neuroplasticity, which in turn worsens sleep and fitness, leading to an increasing number of drug prescriptions. Each intervention creates new problems while failing to address root causes.

Additionally, many service members have a history of childhood trauma. While military service provides structure and purpose, it often adds new layers of trauma. Understanding these pre-existing vulnerabilities helps explain why some veterans struggle more than others.

This chapter examines the biological foundations of veteran mental health struggles that deserve recognition on the path to healing.

————Traumatic brain injury————

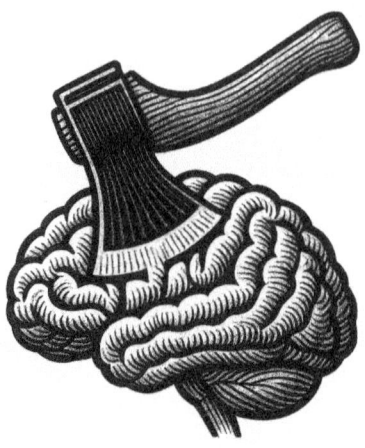

Brain injury that exacerbates mental health disorders is a common consequence of military service.

Blast waves from explosions (e.g., IEDs, artillery), falls, and impact injuries are major contributors to traumatic brain injury in combat zones. Studies show that among soldiers exposed to blasts, around 40 percent show signs of TBI, and as much as 82 percent of combat-TBIs may be blast-related (Institute of Medicine, 2009). Repeated blasts do not produce immediate symptoms of brain injury. Instead, microscopic damage throughout the brain accumulates over time.

Unlike the body's immune system, the brain's immune system lacks an off switch. Consequently, inflammation spreads through the brain like a slow-moving fire, worsening symptoms across years and even decades.

Symptoms of brain injury include:

- Altered personality
- Worsening emotional regulation and impulse control
- Worsening cognitive function (memory, problem-solving, etc.)
- Depression
- Anxiety
- Sleep disturbances

These symptoms illustrate why veterans with brain injuries experience higher rates of PTSD, depression, and suicidal thoughts and why they are often resistant to treatment. When a brain injury coincides with PTSD, factors like moral injury or grief complicate treatment even further. Cognitive challenges resulting from TBI can hinder the ability to process trauma, engage in talk therapy, or benefit from other methods that do not address the underlying neurological issues. Meanwhile, neurological rehabilitation aimed at treating brain injuries may neglect the psychological aspects of a veteran's condition.

Psychedelics and TBI

Research suggests that psychedelics may help address TBI by enhancing brain connectivity and function. Psilocybin can influence blood flow and connectivity in brain regions associated with perception, memory, and attention—areas typically impacted by TBI. Along with its effect on serotonin 2A receptors that regulate mood, psilocybin can assist veterans in tackling rigid thought patterns and depression and anxiety (Palmer, 2025; Blest-Hopley et al., 2025; Velit-Salazar, Shiroma, & Cherian et al., 2024, Kato et al., 2025).

A 2024 Stanford study of special operations forces veterans with TBI showed significant improvements in PTSD, depression, and anxiety following magnesium-ibogaine therapy, with no serious adverse events. (Subjects received magnesium to reduce potential cardiac risks inherent with ibogaine, a psychoactive alkaloid derived from the root bark of the African shrub *Tabernanthe iboga*.) Ibogaine facilitates natural repair mechanisms in key brain regions related to reward, motivation, pleasure, and movement, concurrently addressing neurological and psychological symptoms and damage (Cherian et al., 2024).

While conventional treatments focus on either neurological or psychological symptoms, psychedelics demonstrate the potential to address both. However, it's crucial to highlight that this is a new area of research, and there is a need for more extensive, controlled clinical trials to fully understand the safety and efficacy of these treatments for TBI.

———Physical injury———

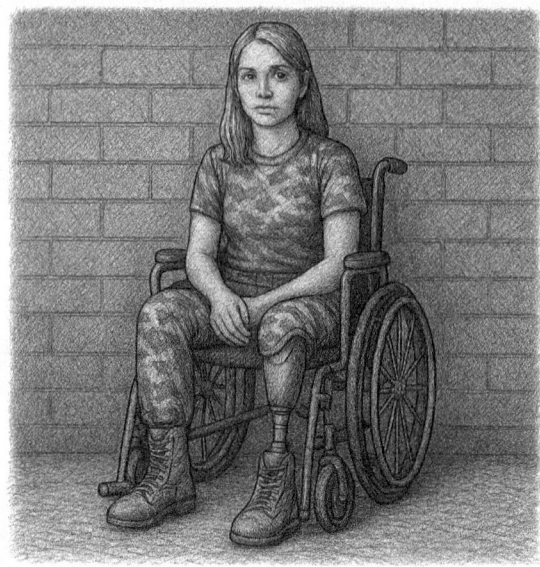

Nearly half of veterans sustain injuries in service that increase the risks of mental health issues.

One out of every ten veterans alive today was seriously injured at some point while serving in the military, and three-quarters of those injuries occurred in combat (Pew Research Center, 2011). These injuries, some severe or permanent, strike at a particularly cruel moment when young service members have pushed their bodies to peak condition, transforming themselves into elite warriors capable of meeting the extreme demands of military service. Injury forces young veterans to completely reimagine their futures, robbing them of possible career, athletic, or recreational pursuits. This sudden shift in identity and capability can spill over into an increased risk of developing PTSD, depression, anxiety, and substance abuse disorders. Research shows higher rates of suicidal ideation and attempts among veterans with physical injuries.

Some of the most devastating are genital injuries, often the result of blast trauma, which can cause lasting sexual dysfunction, infertility, and chronic pain. These injuries not only impact intimate relationships but also strike at the core of identity and self-worth for many veterans. The psychological impact can be as severe as the physical damage, compounding grief, shame, and isolation.

The combination of physical injury and mental health crises creates a vicious cycle in which the two perpetuate one another. Additionally, many veterans face barriers to support systems, rehabilitation services, and effective mental health treatment, worsening their situations.

Psychedelics and injury

While psychedelics have shown promise in facilitating neurological recovery from brain injury, they cannot reverse the damage caused by bodily injury. However, they can assist veterans in processing the grief of lost physical abilities while helping them find new sources of meaning and purpose.

Additionally, emerging research indicates that psychedelic medicines may aid in pain management by modulating serotonin receptors, reducing inflammation, and promoting neuroplasticity in the brain (Yasin, 2024).

The ceremonial context of psychedelic therapy also provides a space where veterans can process their changed relationship with their bodies without the shame or stigma they might feel in traditional medical settings.

———Chemical injury———

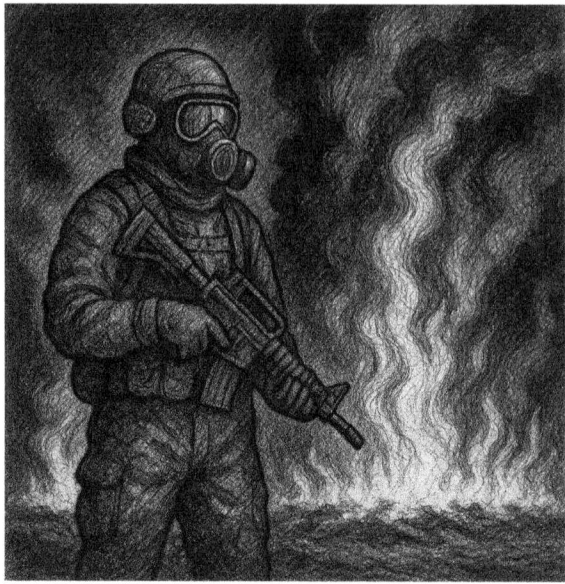

Exposure to toxins promotes chronic health issues and disease and exacerbates mental health disorders, especially when concerns are dismissed by doctors.

Exposure to burn pits, depleted uranium, nerve agents, and environmental contamination are just some of the chemical consequences affecting veteran health, some taking years or even decades to manifest as "unexplained illness."

Many struggle with anxiety and uncertainty about whether their symptoms stem from these exposures, becoming hypervigilant about their health. Being medically dismissed can add to this burden. It wasn't until 2022, with the passage of the Promise to Address Comprehensive Toxics (PACT) Act, that the harms caused by toxic exposures were finally recognized by legislators. Yet many veterans still struggle to navigate the bureaucracy and prove their conditions are service-connected, even as they watch fellow veterans die from exposure-related illnesses.

A veteran dealing with PTSD from combat experiences might find their symptoms exacerbated by chronic respiratory issues from burn pit exposure. Someone struggling with moral injury might have their sense of betrayal deepened by the realization that preventable chemical exposures compromised their health during service.

Psychedelics and chemical injury

As with physical injury, psychedelics can help veterans work through the anxiety and uncertainty about their health while potentially offering relief from some physical symptoms through their anti-inflammatory and neuro-plastic properties.

The ceremonial space of peer support can also help them process the anger, betrayal, and fear surrounding the impact of chemical exposure on their health.

─────Operator Syndrome─────

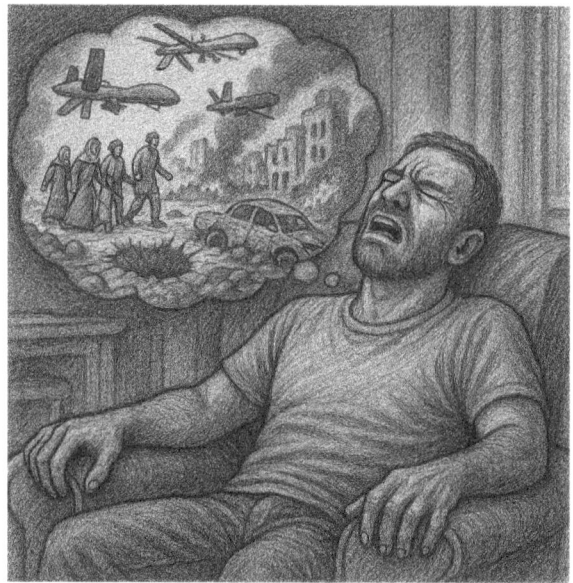

Prolonged states of heightened alertness keep the nervous system locked in fight-or-flight mode, gradually eroding both physical and psychological well-being.

Months or years of existing on high alert, the physical demands of many military roles, repeated blast exposures or head injuries, and traumatic experiences all take a toll on the body. It's no surprise that many veterans leave service with not only mental health challenges but also chronic physical symptoms such as hormonal imbalances, fatigue, insomnia, gut problems, autoimmune disease, chronic inflammation, increased food and chemical sensitivities, and more. Prolonged states of heightened alertness keep the nervous system locked in fight-or-flight mode, gradually eroding both physical and psychological resilience. This cluster of effects is known as Operator Syndrome, a term coined in 2020 by Christopher Frueh, PhD. While Frueh created the term to refer to special operators, operator syndrome can affect anyone subjected to prolonged periods of intense pressure and stress.

The syndrome often manifests as difficulty in "turning off" the high-octane mindset. Veterans may find themselves constantly scanning for threats, struggling to relax in safe environments, or needing to maintain a tactical mindset in everyday situations. The military's culture of toughness further instills the mindset of pushing through a gradual breakdown and refusing to seek support.

Many veterans report feeling unable to fully relax even years after leaving the service, resulting in a state of perpetual exhaustion that affects relationships, work, and overall quality of life.

Clinical symptoms frequently seen in those with Operator Syndrome include:

- Sleep disorders
- Anxiety
- Depression
- Low self-worth and motivation
- Emotional dullness
- Relationship issues
- Low sex hormone levels
- Secondary adrenal insufficiency (low cortisol, or "burnout")
- Weakened immune resilience
- Development of autoimmune disorders
- Increased food or chemical sensitivities
- Gut health issues
- Postural Orthostatic Tachycardia Syndrome (POTS)
- Myalgic Encephalomyelitis/Chronic Fatigue Syndrome (ME/CFS)

Functional medicine approaches to Operator Syndrome

Many veterans have found relief from the symptoms of Operator Syndrome by working within a functional medicine model. Functional medicine differs from conventional medicine in that it seeks the root causes of health problems by examining how all body systems interact, rather than treating each symptom in isolation with a prescription drug. For instance, an untreated brain injury can cause gut problems, or a hormonal imbalance can trigger an autoimmune disease. Functional medicine practitioners examine how stress, diet, sleep, and environment impact health and tailor a protocol to an individual's unique physiological needs. A pharmaceutical approach cannot treat many of the underlying mechanisms of Operator Syndrome.

Examples of interventions include supporting cortisol rhythms, repairing gut barrier integrity and gut microbiome health, reducing inflammation, supporting cellular energy production, balancing hormones, implementing stress reduction strategies, etc.

Psychedelics and Operator Syndrome

Psychedelic work may help calm an overactive nervous system, allowing some to relax for the first time in many years. Some veterans, particularly those who grew up with trauma, report feeling safe for the first time in their lives during a psychedelic journey. This can help them learn how to practice releasing the constant need for control and hypervigilance in their daily lives.

By promoting neuroplasticity and resetting default mode patterns in the brain, psychedelics may help consistently "wired" veterans develop healthier responses to everyday environments. The ceremonial context of psychedelic healing can also assist veterans in addressing the underlying traumas associated with Operator Syndrome, teaching them how to modulate their responses based on actual threats versus perceived ones.

————Neuroplastic disorder————

Sometimes, a person makes great strides in their mental health journey, but their nervous system is still stuck in fight-or-flight mode, which may contribute to chronic pain or health symptoms. The culprit is neuroplasticity, the brain's ability to reorganize itself by forming new neural connections. Neuroplasticity can be positive, such as learning a new skill, or negative, such as developing bad habits or becoming hyper-efficient at detecting danger when there is none.

Prolonged exposure to life-threatening or severely stressful situations creates neural pathways that prioritize threat detection. While effective in combat zones, this wiring becomes problematic when the nervous system continues to trigger alarm responses in the absence of a threat.

This neurological hypersensitivity to stimuli is often referred to as *neuroplastic disorder*. It is characterized by one's nervous system developing exaggerated reactivity to pain, light, sound, touch, and other stimuli. While the mental health consequences of neuroplastic disorder are better understood (PTSD, for example), what's lesser known is that this dynamic can also contribute to chronic pain and health symptoms.

Symptoms and disorders that can be perpetuated by neuroplastic disorder:

- Fibromyalgia
- Chronic regional pain syndrome (CRPS)
- Irritable bowel syndrome
- Tension headaches and migraines
- Temporomandibular disorders
- Multiple chemical sensitivities
- Multiple food sensitivities
- Some forms of chronic fatigue syndrome

Neuroplastic disorder is like a doorbell that rings louder and longer each time it's pressed, releasing inflammatory compounds that further activate the nervous system in a vicious cycle. The result is that it reacts strongly even to mild triggers.

This can explain why some veterans develop chronic health and pain struggles. This isn't to say structural damage or metabolic disorders shouldn't be treated. However, sometimes, symptoms may persist or become over-exaggerated in proportion to the physiological insult due to neuroplastic disorder.

The good news is that various approaches offer promise. While psychedelics aren't necessary for these approaches to work, they create windows of optimal neuroplasticity that make neuroplastic therapies a great complement.

For instance, pain reprocessing therapy (PRT) targets the brain circuits that misinterpret bodily sensations as threatening, amplifying pain or other symptoms. This approach helps people recognize when pain or other symptoms are driven by neural pathways rather than tissue damage. Through guided exercises, a care recipient teaches their nervous system to better distinguish between dangerous and safe sensations, building physiological resilience and reducing symptoms.

Integration with psychedelic therapy
Many people find significant relief using neuroplastic approaches without psychedelics. However, those who choose to work with psychedelics find that they complement neuroplastic therapy.

Psychedelics create temporary periods of heightened neuroplasticity during which the brain becomes exceptionally receptive to forming new connections. This provides an ideal opportunity to introduce new interpretations of bodily sensations before neural pathways have re-solidified. A person with chronic pain or health symptoms can maximize these windows of opportunity with challenges that rewire deep-seated threat responses that arise from neuroplastic disorder.

———Worsening fitness———

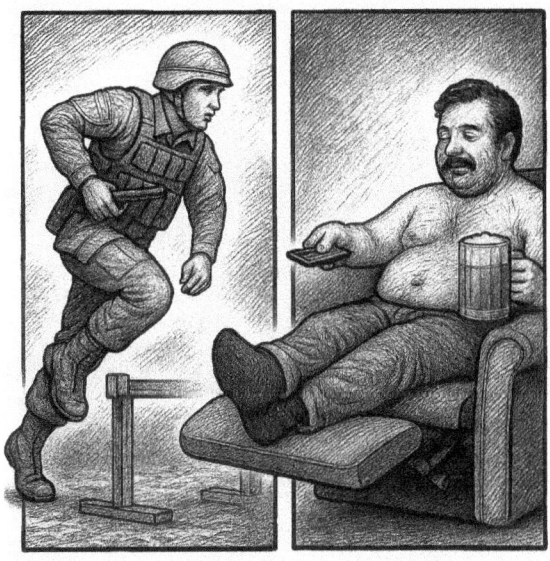

After years of maintaining peak physical condition in the military, many veterans struggle with the abrupt loss of fitness once they return to civilian life.

Veterans who once prided themselves on their peak physical condition may struggle with weight gain and a decline in strength and endurance after exiting military service. Research shows that regular exercise can profoundly support mood and mental well-being, meaning this physical decline can trigger or worsen depression and anxiety.

The problem is compounded when chronic pain, joint injuries, and other physical limitations acquired in service are involved, especially in those whose sense of self was closely tied to their physical capabilities.

The loss of the military's structured physical training environment also means losing a source of social connection and stress relief that many service members rely on for mental health maintenance.

Psychedelics and fitness
Psychedelics don't directly impact physical fitness, but many people find a renewed devotion to improving their health when processing their mental health issues through psychedelic healing. Responding to the body's needs for regular vigorous activity is just one of many ways people nurture the self-love reawakened in psychedelic healing.

———Substance abuse———

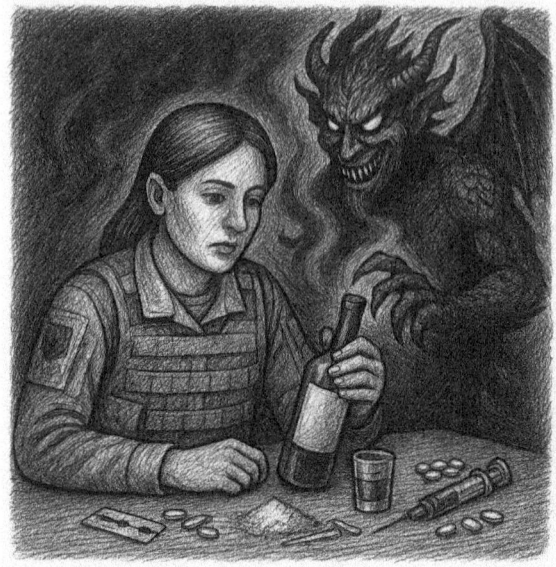

Substance abuse develops when one tries to medicate their symptoms.
It's short-term relief and a long-term worsening of mental health.

Substance abuse is a particularly insidious response to mental health challenges, offering a short-term "emotional anesthesia" with devastating long-term consequences. Veterans face significantly higher rates of substance use disorders than civilians (National Institute on Drug Abuse [NIDA], 2020).

In a desperate attempt at relief, they may turn to alcohol or drugs to cope with PTSD symptoms, moral injury, TBI symptoms, or unprocessed grief from losing comrades. It's a deal with the devil, as substance abuse often worsens mental health and causes additional problems like losing relationships and jobs.

Traditional addiction treatment programs may not adequately address the underlying trauma, moral injury, or grief driving the substance use. Meanwhile, mental health treatments may be less effective if substance use continues to interfere with the processing and integration of traumatic experiences.

Psychedelics and substance abuse

Psychedelics appear to modulate the same neurotransmitter systems involved in addiction while promoting neuroplasticity that helps restructure destructive patterns of thought and behavior. Psychedelic work must be supported with ample preparation and integration, as well as with changes to one's home and social life in a way that promotes sobriety.

Ibogaine, in particular, shows potential for treating substance use disorders, especially opiate addiction. Studies have shown that ibogaine can significantly reduce withdrawal symptoms and drug cravings by modulating neurotransmitter systems in the brain's reward and motivation circuits. It simultaneously helps veterans process the root causes of their addictions. Due to ibogaine's potential cardiac risks, careful medical screening and monitoring are essential.

————Pre-service trauma and PTSD————

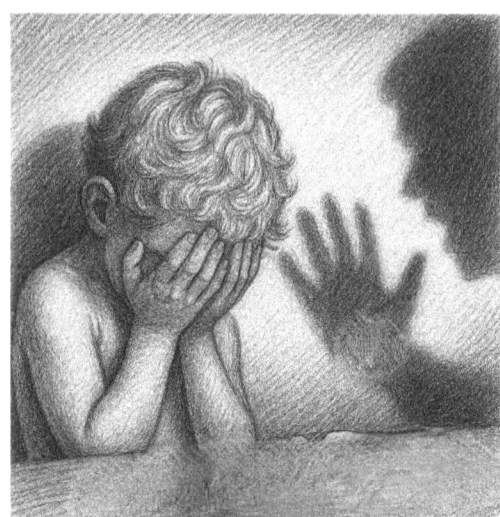

Compared to civilians, veterans are more likely to report early childhood abuse and trauma.

Solely focusing on military-related trauma may miss crucial pieces of the puzzle. Many veterans enter service already suffering from past trauma or PTSD stemming from childhood abuse or interpersonal violence. Research indicates that, compared to civilians, veterans are more likely to report childhood sexual abuse, childhood physical abuse, and exposure to domestic violence prior to entering military service (Rossi et al., 2025). Some enlist simply to escape abuse at home, with this pre-existing trauma compounding the risk of developing PTSD, depression, and substance use disorders from combat or military experiences in what researchers call posttraumatic decline.

Certain factors before deployment have been shown to help buffer these effects, such as a good ability to plan, focus, and control impulses, and strong social support networks. However, pre-existing psychiatric conditions and limited social support can amplify the effects of trauma acquired during service.

Psychedelics and pre-existing trauma

We have frequently seen veterans process early childhood and pre-existing traumas instead of their service-related trauma in their first psychedelic retreat. If they continue to work with psychedelics, confronting their military-related trauma often comes later. The psyche instinctively knows to work through traumas in an order that makes sense for optimal healing.

———Polypharmacy———

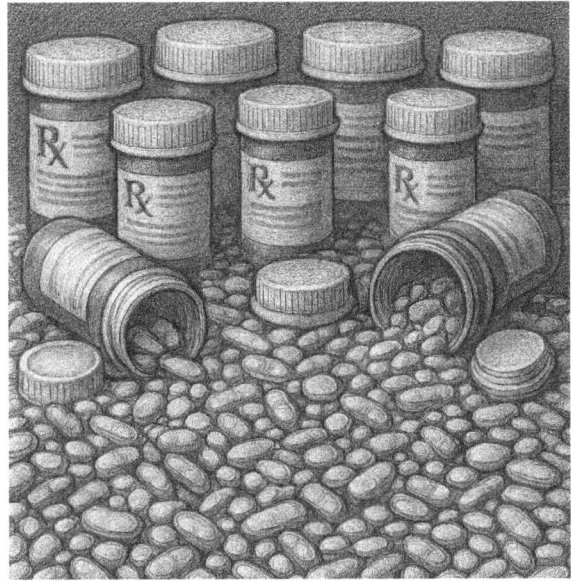

Veterans are often prescribed multiple psychiatric medications.

Almost half of veterans admitted for PTSD treatment are taking five or more medications simultaneously, roughly three times the rate seen in U.S. adults overall (Raut et al., 2025). We have met veterans taking *up to a dozen psychiatric drugs*.

The situation becomes particularly dangerous with benzodiazepines, commonly prescribed for anxiety and sleep issues. While they provide short-term relief, they carry serious risks of dependency and severe withdrawal symptoms that include extreme anxiety, insomnia, and even seizures.

Multiple medications often interact in unpredictable ways, leading to new symptoms that might be mistaken for additional mental health issues. This can trigger a cascade where more medications are prescribed to address side effects from existing ones. Veterans with complex health needs or limited access to coordinated care face the highest risks of dangerous drug interactions and adverse effects.

Worst of all, medication alone—and especially multiple medications—fails to address the root causes of veteran mental health challenges and may even impede healing.

Psychedelics and polypharmacy

Addressing veterans' prescription drug use is outside the scope of HHP. However, we ask veterans who want to participate in a psychedelic retreat to work with their doctor to safely wean off their psychiatric medications before attending a retreat.

Of particular concern are antidepressants, antipsychotics, and mood stabilizers. Their interactions with psychedelics can be unpredictable and potentially dangerous.

SSRIs (selective serotonin reuptake inhibitors) and other antidepressants typically need to be carefully tapered under medical supervision before participating in psychedelic therapy. Similarly, benzodiazepines can significantly diminish the effects of psychedelics while also carrying their own risks during withdrawal.

Veterans taking multiple psychiatric medications may need several months of careful medication management before participating in psychedelic therapy.

Before attending a psychedelic retreat, it's crucial to:

- Disclose all medications to retreat organizers
- Work with your doctor to safely taper off psychiatric medications before a retreat
- Allow sufficient time for any medication adjustments
- Understand that some medications or psychiatric conditions (such as schizophrenia or bipolar disorder) may make psychedelic therapy unsuitable

---

CHAPTER 6

COMMUNAL INJURY

While psychological and biological wounds impact veteran mental health, social wounds, or what might be called "communal injuries," also play a significant role. Military service creates an intense sense of belonging and shared mission. When that bond is severed, many veterans face a profound loss of community, compounded by distance from the camaraderie, humor, and purpose that once anchored their daily lives. The return to civilian life often brings culture shock, stigmatization, and pathologization.

These pressures strain marriages, friendships, and family ties, sometimes worsening relationships just when support is most needed, thrusting many veterans into isolation and loneliness that magnifies their other challenges.

This chapter examines how loss of connection and meaning, civilian misunderstandings, and social stigma interact to create communal injury, factors that must be acknowledged and addressed for genuine healing to occur.

Loss of community and
ceremonial aspects of service

To understand the challenges modern veterans face, it helps to look at the history of military culture, writes Nathan J. Hogan, PhD, author of *Martial Culture in the Lifeways of U.S. Service members and Veterans* (Hogan, 2024). What Hogan calls "martial culture" traces back to humanity's earliest need to survive against predators and hostile intruders. The notion of the "civilian" is a relatively recent development, first appearing among a small ruling class before becoming the norm in industrialized, first-world nations.

Military service reshapes identity, with basic training serving not only as job preparation but also as an initiation into an entirely new culture. In earlier times, this transition was reinforced by rituals and ceremonies rooted in humanity's oldest traditions, practices designed to integrate warriors into their communities and give meaning to their service. The Greeks, Romans, feudal Japanese, Norse, and indigenous cultures passed down these frameworks through generations to help warriors understand their roles and place in society. Today, the corporatization of the military has largely stripped away such traditions, leaving recruits without these time-tested pathways of integration.

Military culture centers on service and the sacrifice of the individual for the collective. As the saying goes, "There are those who serve and those who are served." While reasons for joining can range from practical considerations to a noble calling, at the core lies the commitment to protecting the broader society. This warrior identity extends well beyond the battlefield and, for many, endures long after discharge, shaping how service members see themselves and their place in the world.

One of the least understood aspects of martial culture is what Hogan calls the "ecstatic warrior experience," which refers to the transcendent flow states commonly experienced during training and combat. While recognized and even honored in ancient warrior-shamanic traditions, modern recruits lack a similar cultural reference point for these experiences. They tend to hide or downplay the ecstatic state, fearing pathologization by a clinical culture that has long since distanced itself from natural spiritual states.

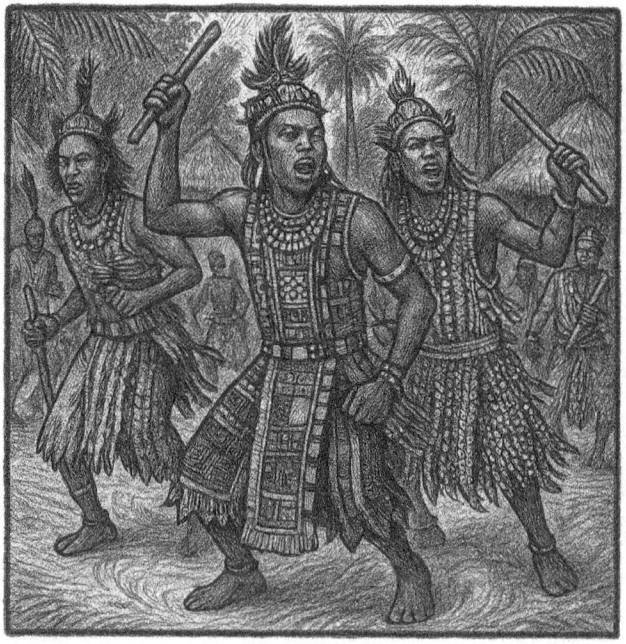

The "ecstatic warrior experience" was long understood to be integral to the military experience prior to the modernization of warfare.

This mirrors what Sebastian Junger discovered among Mende warriors of

Sierra Leone, who described combat as making the heart "heat up," transforming fighters into an altered state where they "literally became someone else." The rhythmic movement, chanting, and extreme physical challenges of training also dissolve one's identity into a collective altered state.

While the Mende recognized this transformation as a natural part of warfare, modern military culture provides no such framework for understanding these profound shifts in consciousness (Junger, 2016).

The modern denial of such spiritual significance abandons the service member to enter and exit these states without guidance, integration, or completion, unlike traditional Mende culture, which acknowledged that the "moral excesses of the battlefield" need not be carried home when properly understood and integrated.

Instead, modern society tends to view veterans through a binary lens: either damaged or heroic, overlooking the complex reality of military culture.

How psychedelics help veterans integrate
Psychedelic-assisted therapy for veterans provides meaningful transition rituals for integration back into society, healing rites among the safety of peers, and the acknowledgment of their evolving cultural identity and spiritual heritage.

These therapeutic approaches, particularly in veteran-specific settings with trained veteran facilitators, provide the ritual frameworks and ceremonial spaces that Hogan identifies as crucial for veteran healing.

Unlike traditional therapy that may pathologize these experiences, psychedelic journeys provide a setting to process and honor the warrior aspect of identity. The history of psychedelic ceremonies parallels that of warrior traditions, both of which center on transformation. The veteran group setting creates space to speak without fear of judgment or pathologization, to reconnect with the positive aspects of military culture, to process its traumatic elements without shame, and to remember one's place in an ancient lineage.

This addresses what Hogan identifies as a crucial need: maintaining a connection to military identity while adapting to civilian society. These approaches don't seek to "fix" veterans or rehabilitate or suppress this identity. Instead, they provide tools for integrating this identity while building bridges to civilian life.

Just as traditional warriors used ceremonial contexts to "control the tempo of the storm," veteran psychedelic therapy provides similar transformative experiences to help them process the intense states they experienced in combat and training.

While modern military culture often leaves service members to navigate these states alone, veteran-specific psychedelic therapy offers a culturally appropriate container in which participants can find meaning, resilience, and connection.

————Loss of purpose and prestige————

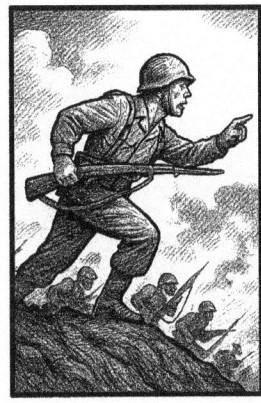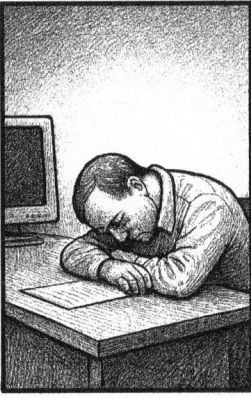

After military service, a civilian job can feel hollow and purposeless.

The transition from military service to civilian life marks a new chapter in life that may feel suddenly hollow for some. Soldiers are on the frontline of geopolitical events, giving them a tangible sense of purpose. This is especially true for those who strongly believed in their mission or served in a high level of engagement, such as in special operations. Back in a corporate or academic environment, life can feel purposeless and meaningless.

Veterans may also lose their reputation, rank, or distinction. During combat or service, they may have successfully led teams, protected comrades, and made critical decisions. They understood their role in supporting the larger mission, whether they were maintaining aircraft, coordinating logistics, or leading combat operations. Uniform insignia and medals tell a straightforward story of achievement and sacrifice that other service members instantly understand and honor.

Back home, these life-and-death skills may be seen as irrelevant or even problematic, something the veteran feels they must hide. A Navy SEAL or senior NCO now finds themselves in an entry-level position where the stakes feel trivially low compared to their military responsibilities. Contrast this to most soldiers throughout history, like the Iroquois, who were still relied upon for hunting, fishing, and participation in everyday life after each battle. Their warrior identity was preserved and valued during peacetime, not set aside. Many modern veterans, by contrast, struggle to translate their hard-earned battle skills into meaningful civilian roles.

Losing this clearly defined purpose after separation from service can create a devastating void. Hogan notes, "The service member-turned-veteran is now a stranger in a strange land."

Veterans often report feeling stripped of their identity, struggling to find meaning, and questioning their value and role in society. This loss of purpose and prestige is a legitimate challenge, not a personal failure to adapt.

Psychedelics and purpose

Psychedelic healing experiences can help veterans honor rather than suppress or pathologize their warrior identity and the meaningful aspects of their military experience. Additionally, many who undergo profound healing feel compelled to train as a coach or facilitator to bring that healing to others, giving them renewed purpose. Or they connect with a newfound passion and their own personal evolution.

—————Loss of humorous interactions—————

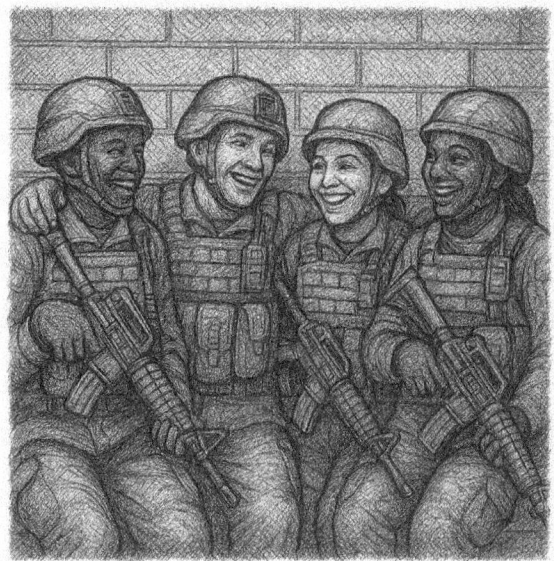

Civilian life typically does not offer the same degree of gallows humor.

The unique humor that develops among service members, characterized as dark, irreverent, and incomprehensible to outsiders, serves as a survival mechanism and a means of bonding. The ability to laugh in the face of danger, hardship, and darkness is a fundamental coping mechanism integral to military culture.

Service members can process trauma, grief, and fear through jokes that would shock most civilians, yet serve as a vital pressure release valve. As a result, veterans may have to suppress their dark humor, which feels like another aspect of cultural exile and the loss of emotional processing and collegial intimacy.

At the same time, it's crucial to recognize that humor can be an unproductive crutch that stands in the way of healing. It can also become a form of bullying or cruelty.

Psychedelics and humor

While psychedelic healing requires intense personal work, it also brings bouts of deep joy, playfulness, and levity, often for the first time in years for many people. Journeying alongside peers creates a space for many light-hearted and humorous moments. The fantastical and sometimes absurd nature of the psychedelic mystical experience offers ample material for humor.

————Civilian culture shock————

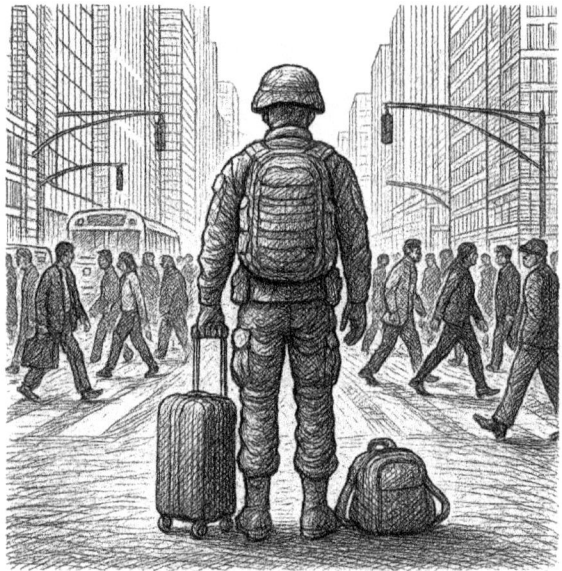

Civilian life can be a culture shock after service and combat, leaving one feeling alienated.

When veterans leave the military, they don't just change jobs. Military discharge plunges one into profound culture shock and alienation that few civilians understand. It often comes as a surprise to veterans and their loved ones alike.

Military life emphasizes collective goals, sacrifice, and blunt communication. Civilian culture, in contrast, prioritizes individuality, comfort, and communication mired in unspoken cues and hidden meanings. Veterans must learn to temper their directness and navigate complex hierarchies, such as office politics. This can leave a veteran feeling perpetually out of place.

Civilian culture shock also reflects the clash between our evolutionary tribal heritage and the isolationism of modern society. Technological advances and material conveniences have come at the cost of our innate design for collective purpose and connection, which military service recreates and civilian life strips away again.

As such, service members return to a civilian world at war with itself and ruled by what Junger notes as "a level of contempt usually reserved for enemies in wartime, except that now it's applied to our fellow citizens" (Junger, 2016).

Psychedelics and civilian culture shock

Veterans often report that their psychedelic journeys helped them gain new perspectives on civilian culture without feeling pressured to abandon their military identity. Instead of feeling trapped between two worlds, this can help them learn to move more fluidly between military and civilian identities.

———The pathologization of veterans———

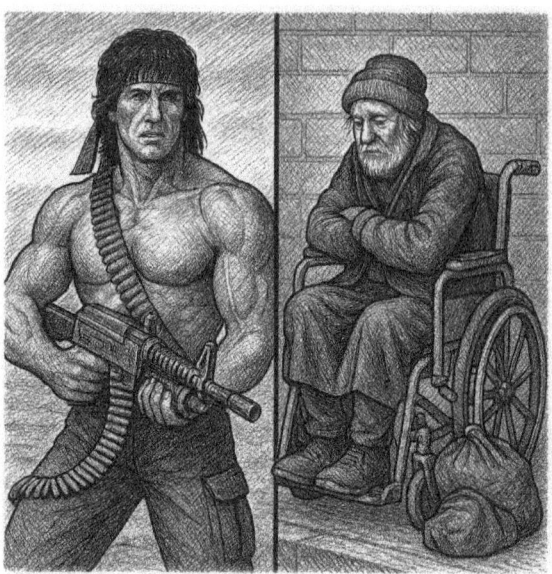

Veterans tend to be either mythologized or vilified by a civilian culture that is largely ignorant of military service.

Rather than recognizing military service as an enduring cultural tradition, civilians often view veterans through a lens of damage, dysfunction, and victimhood. Despite good intentions, the healthcare system can frame military service as aberrant or maladaptive, something to be "fixed" so one can fit in.

The qualities that make a service member effective are often perceived as traits to be eliminated rather than integrated into the civilian world. This puts veterans in a bind: they must either suppress their military identity or risk being viewed as psychologically damaged. According to Hogan, this results in a form of cultural erasure disguised as treatment, where the goal becomes stripping away the military identity rather than helping veterans integrate their military experiences into civilian life.

This pathologization fails to recognize that many veterans' struggles stem from cultural displacement rather than psychological damage, requiring cultural reintegration rather than solely clinical intervention.

Additionally, the medical model often encourages veterans to see themselves as victims, a stark contrast to their active-duty mindset, where "the passivity of victimhood can get them killed" (Junger, 2016). Traditional tribal cultures viewed combat as part of a maturation process, and returning warriors were considered integral to their society, not outsiders who needed to be pitied or fixed. While symptoms of alienation may mirror those of PTSD, the psychological displacement that comes from losing one's tribal connections and warrior identity is being misdiagnosed as a clinical disorder rather than a natural response to losing both tribal bonds and meaningful societal purpose.

Psychedelics and pathologization

Unlike conventional mental health treatments that may seek to "correct" military cultural traits, psychedelic experiences in veteran-specific settings honor the warrior identity while facilitating its healthy integration into civilian life.

———Stigma of war———

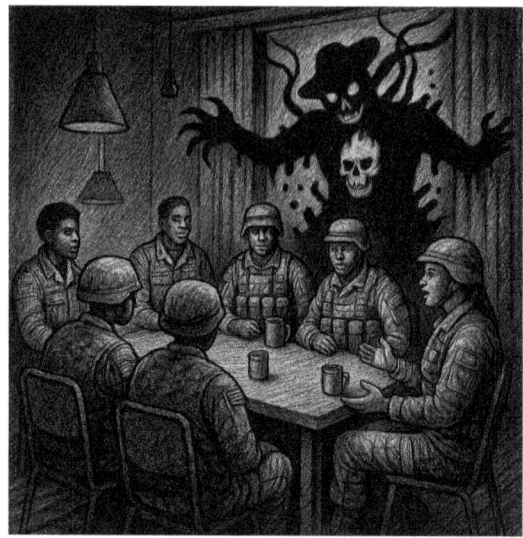

Veterans are often stigmatized in civilian culture.

In contrast to historic cultures, many modern Westerners view military service through a lens of shame or moral failure, creating a paradox where veterans serve a culture that often stigmatizes them. Veterans return home to find that the skills and mindset that made them effective in service are now viewed with suspicion or pity. This can push veterans to suppress parts of their identity, leading to feelings of alienation.

Veterans are not victims. They are members of society who have experienced the darker sides of humanity. While we all hope for more peace, there has nevertheless been a need for a warrior class since the dawn of civilization. Participation in that world carries unique traumas. Every person chose to enter this role for their own reasons, suffered wounds as a consequence, and deserves access to healing. They are called service members for a reason.

Psychedelics and the stigma of war
Veteran-specific psychedelic retreats create spaces where participants can openly discuss combat experiences, dark humor, pride in their service, and transcendent states without fear of judgment or misunderstanding.

Rather than trying to "fix" veterans or strip away their military identity, psychedelic healing can help them honor this aspect of themselves while building bridges to civilian life.

By integrating their warrior experiences into a broader understanding of human nature and conflict, they find peace and pride in their service background and the strength and wisdom it has given them.

————Worsening relationships————

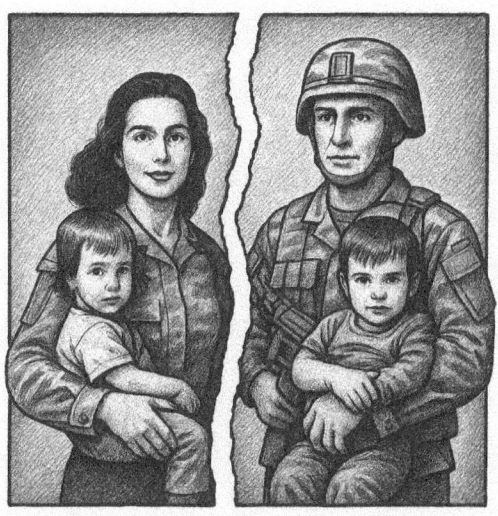

The mental health challenges veterans face can strain and break relationships.

Many veterans with mental health challenges experience strained or broken relationships with partners, families, children, or coworkers. Internal chaos and dysfunction inevitably spill over into these connections, creating a cruel paradox: the veteran most needs support from their closest relationships, yet those very people may be driven away by mistreatment, unhealthy dynamics, or safety concerns. This loss of connection deepens the veteran's isolation, shame, and sense of unworthiness.

Men in particular avoid seeking help due to perceived weakness, or they withdraw from their partners. However, research indicates that engaging partners in the healing journey yields better outcomes. For veterans experiencing homelessness or dealing with military sexual trauma, these challenges become even more acute, with mental health and relationship difficulties compounding one another.

Psychedelics and relationships
Many veterans have found that psychedelic healing and MDMA-assisted therapy help them examine their relationship patterns from a more neutral and compassionate perspective, gaining insight into the role their trauma

plays. The ability to do this free from self-hatred, shame, anger, or a sense of victimhood frees the individual to work toward a fresh start.

Veteran peer support is particularly crucial in this process. When veterans share their experiences with other veterans, they rediscover their capacity for authentic connections, an escape from isolation, and the importance of being accepted and understood. This peer support is also vital during the post-journey integration period.

Psychedelic retreats for veteran spouses

Due to the impact of mental health issues on primary relationships, HHP began offering retreats for veteran spouses. We recognized that excluding partners from the process was unfair to them and ineffective for veterans, especially after years of conflict and strain. Returning to a home environment filled with resentment or animosity can hinder a veteran's progress, as their partner, who has been experiencing secondary trauma from the veteran, did not have the same opportunity for breakthrough insights.

Sharing psychedelic healing work can help partners gain a deeper understanding of one another while creating new foundations for communication and intimacy. Couples often report breaking through communication barriers and gaining a deeper understanding of their partner's perspective.

The healing potential extends to the entire family system, creating ripple effects that benefit veterans' children and extended family.

By creating spaces where veterans and their partners can heal together, psychedelic therapy offers hope for breaking cycles of trauma that often pass through generations of veteran families.

———Isolation———

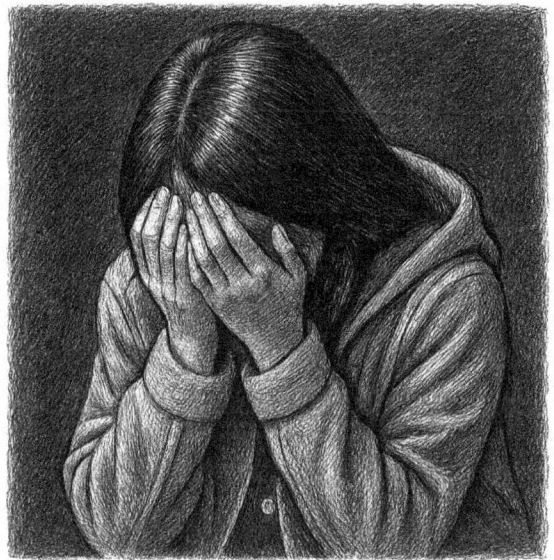

Isolation is a common and potentially risky problem for veterans struggling with mental health issues.

Isolation is a common and potentially risky problem for veterans struggling with mental health issues. They find themselves suddenly cut off from the intense bonds of military service, thrust into a civilian world that can't understand or relate to their experiences, and sometimes estranged from their loved ones.

Additionally, those with depression, PTSD, and other issues often withdraw from social connections, which in turn worsens psychological well-being. The COVID-19 pandemic particularly impacted veterans struggling with isolation by fracturing existing support networks.

Studies show that among trauma-exposed individuals, lack of social support is a very strong predictor of increased PTSD symptom severity—often as significant or nearly as influential as how severe the trauma was itself (Dworkin et al., 2018; Fares-Otero et al., 2024). This means a veteran with relatively mild trauma exposure could develop long-term PTSD simply due to insufficient social support. The research emphasizes that veterans need connections that understand and honor their military experience while helping them bridge the gap to civilian life.

Psychedelics and isolation

Psychedelics are well known for reawakening our innate wiring for deep communal bonds. Such bonds are challenging to realize in an industrialized world built around individualism.

Unlike traditional one-on-one therapy settings, veteran psychedelic retreats create an immediate sense of belonging through shared military experience and understanding. Veterans often report feeling truly seen and understood for the first time since leaving service.

The psychedelic experience can help them understand how trauma may have led them to withdraw from relationships, recognize their need for connection, and reduce the fear and hypervigilance that may have kept them isolated.

The process of preparation, journeying, and integration with a group of peers provides a controlled environment where veterans can practice vulnerability and rebuild trust among others in a similar state. This shared vulnerability, combined with the profound nature of psychedelic experiences, often creates lasting bonds between retreat participants. Veterans then learn to translate their retreat experiences into practical skills for building and maintaining relationships in their daily lives.

CHAPTER 7

THE HIDDEN WAR: MILITARY SEXUAL TRAUMA

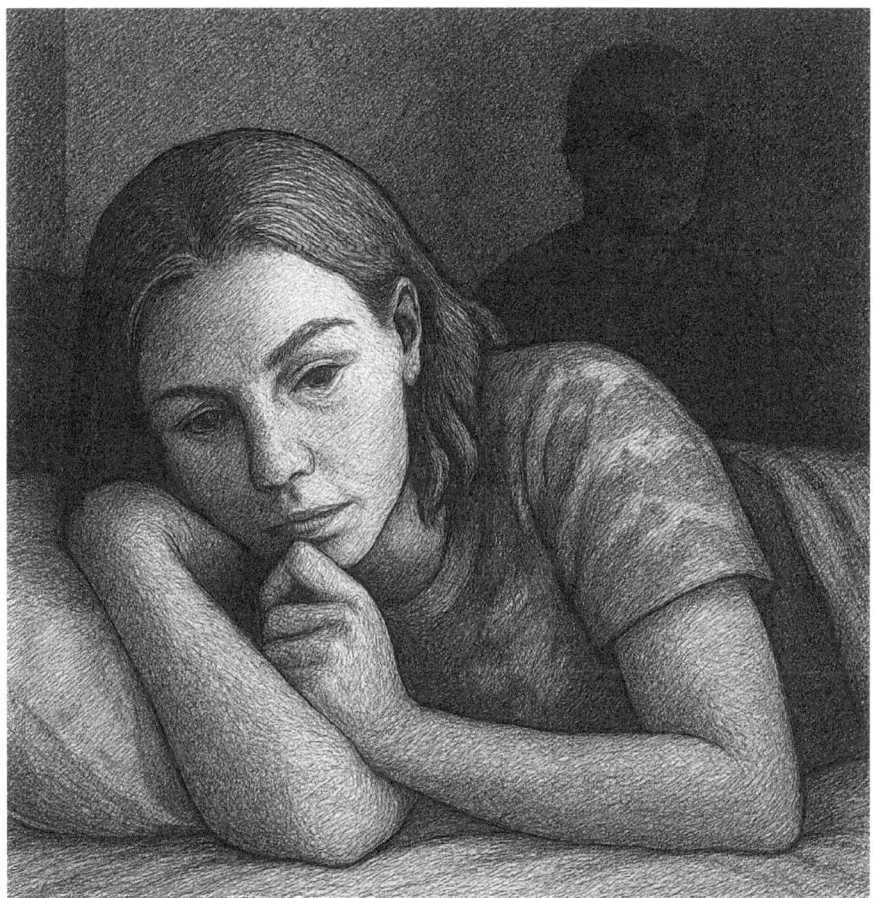

Military sexual trauma affects both women and men, raising the risk of PTSD and other mental health disorders. Victims are often retaliated against for reporting it.

Military sexual trauma (MST) represents one of the most devastating betrayals a service member can endure—violations by those they are trained to trust with their lives. MST proves more predictive of PTSD than other types of military trauma, including combat exposure.

More than half of female recruits report persistent sexual harassment, sometimes to debilitating degrees. Men account for up to half of all MST cases because of their larger numbers in the armed forces, but women are at a far greater risk by population. MST is significantly underreported, with only about 33 percent of women and less than 2 percent of men disclosing their experiences, rates that research suggests is lower than civilian reporting rates (U.S. Department of Veterans Affairs, n.d.).

Compounding the trauma is the frequent retaliation against victims. Those who report assault or harassment are often met with blame, ostracism, stalled promotion, demotion, bullying, or reassignment to undesirable posts. Perpetrators are frequently superiors with direct influence over the victim's career, creating a powerful deterrent to reporting. This culture of retaliation not only warns others to stay silent but also forces many victims to continue serving alongside their attackers, enduring ongoing harassment or assault.

Experts suggest the military's hypermasculine, hierarchical, and "survival of the fittest" culture, where hazing often turns into assault, fosters MST. Additionally, a frequently toxic and unethical chain of command further supports MST. This betrays the true warrior ethos of respecting and protecting team members.

———A unique psychological wound———

MST is a betrayal that is uniquely piercing because it comes from a fellow squad member who is meant to have your back in a life-or-death situation, and victims are under institutional pressure to stay quiet. MST compounds other traumas acquired during service or pre-service, exacerbating psychological injury. Failing to seek help for fear of retaliation compounds the symptoms over time.

While the military population already faces higher rates of PTSD and mental health challenges compared to civilians, MST survivors show even more severe outcomes.

———Psychedelics and MST———

Survivors often struggle to put their experiences into words or have become emotionally disconnected from their trauma, making conventional therapy difficult. Psychedelic- and MDMA-assisted therapies can help them access and work through painful memories while maintaining a sense of physical and emotional safety.

For male survivors who face cultural stigma and shame around MST, psychedelic experiences can help them process their trauma in a setting free from profoundly ingrained shame and silence.

In veteran-specific retreats, survivors can better process trauma among peers who understand the toxic aspects of military culture that silenced them during service.

Veteran voices

Marine Officer Lauren Connally's story illustrates the journey many female service members face. From a close-knit family of veterans, she joined Texas A&M's ROTC program but was immediately met with exclusion by all but a dozen of her male peers, who she grew to trust. Ultimately, however, it was one of those "buddies" who sexually assaulted her, placing her in an impossible position: report and potentially lose everything, or remain silent.

"Here I was around all these misogynistic men that wouldn't even talk to me, and yet someone that I thought I could trust, who was within my unit, is the one that ultimately betrayed me that way," Connally recalls. "He was also a leader within our class. I understand now that there was a lot of fear of losing everything I had worked so hard to gain."

For Connally, choosing silence wasn't cowardice but survival. "I never reported it. I never mourned it. I never acknowledged it other than to beat myself up and say, 'I'm never allowing that to happen again.'"

MST became routine throughout her career and three Iraq deployments, requiring constant hypervigilance. Men would ask for sexual favors if she needed assistance, and routinely break into her quarters while she was sleeping to try to coerce her into sex. She learned that she had to set boundaries and protect herself because the men she served with couldn't be trusted to respect professional boundaries.

This constant hypervigilance led to autoimmune issues, emotional numbness, and deep shame. "I carried the shame of what happened to me all alone, as if it were my fault. I didn't tell my family. I didn't tell my peers. I didn't tell my leadership. I didn't tell anybody."

After leaving the Marines in 2007, Connally spent ten years pretending her military career never happened, even cutting ties with Marine friends. She began reacknowledging that part of herself when her youngest female cousin expressed interest in enlisting.

"She asked for my mentorship and I didn't want her to experience the negative aspects I saw in service," Connally said. "I wanted my story to be wisdom for vigilance, not a deterrent from serving."

She began cognitive processing therapy through the VA, which helped her confront her trauma narratives. "It wasn't that I should have locked my door; it's that he should not have ever come into my room, locked my door, and assaulted me," she explained. "But it takes a lot to be able to say that." Yet she continued struggling with emotional numbness.

At HHP's first U.S.-based psilocybin retreat in Bend, Oregon, Connally finally processed her grief with "profound emotional release." The psychedelic experience helped her reconnect with both painful and positive memories from her military service, including recognizing the good men who had supported her. This balance helped her emerge with "a beautiful emotional neutrality" toward her traumatic memories.

Connally emphasized the importance of proper support throughout the psychedelic experience: "If we're bringing things out of ourselves that are big like this, we have to make sure we're taking measures to integrate them in a way that's really healthy."

CHAPTER 8

NAVIGATING A POLARIZED CULTURE: MARGINALIZED VETERANS

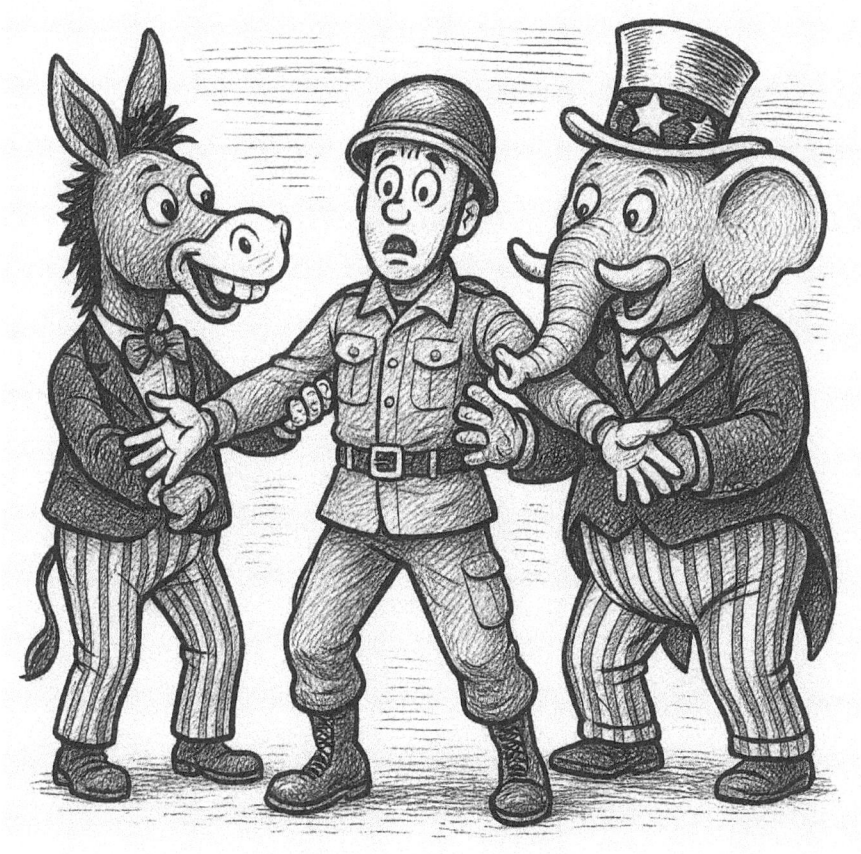

HHP operates on results, not ideology, identity, or politics.

As a psychedelic organization that serves veterans, we sometimes find ourselves caught in the fray of a politically polarized society.

HHP operates on results, not ideology, identity, or politics. This means that newcomers may be grouped into retreats based on what they have in common, such as women, sexual orientation, people of color, veteran spouses, veterans with military sexual trauma, or other communities. This has repelled some veterans for fear of joining a "woke" organization that excludes them for their religious or political beliefs.

We understand this concern, but in our experience, it's easier for veterans new to psychedelics to let down their guard and access greater healing when among peers of similar backgrounds. This is why HHP was created in the first place: to provide veterans with a space to process their experiences more openly among one another than they'd be able to do among civilians.

For instance, a black Army mechanic will have had a different service experience than a white Navy SEAL. A queer Marine who served during "Don't Ask, Don't Tell" may have different struggles than their straight counterpart, and women will have had different experiences than men. It's easier for people to let their guard down around those of a similar background. This subjectivity can also apply to those who served within a specific branch or people from the same unit.

However, if a veteran continues to work with psychedelics, we encourage them to move into more diverse groups. One of the primary lessons of psychedelic work is that all humans grapple with similar core issues; we are all more alike than different. Experiencing this firsthand can help some people release the belief that no one understands them.

Additionally, psychedelic healing often enables individuals to better navigate the "grey areas" within a polarized society. In reality, black-and-white thinking is frequently a symptom of trauma. Real life exists on a wide spectrum and demands mental flexibility.

Nevertheless, we remain emphatic that veterans experience their initial breakthroughs in a veteran-specific setting. This ensures they do not have to self-censor to avoid shocking civilians with their combat experiences or feel they need to keep their guard up.

Everyone who served deserves access to effective help.

LGBTQ+ service members
and multiple layers of trauma

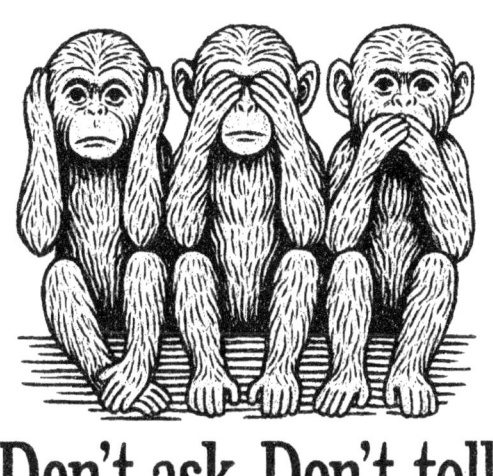

Don't ask. Don't tell.

Military service has historically carried greater risks
for LGBTQ+ members who are outed.

Many LGBTQ+ veterans who served under the "Don't Ask, Don't Tell" policy were essentially penalized for their identity, disclosure of which would have been career-ending. This forced untold numbers of service members to hide a fundamental aspect of their identity, perpetuating a cycle of enforced secrecy and shame.

Service has historically carried greater risks for LGBTQ+ members who are outed. Research shows they are twice as likely to experience military sexual trauma (MST) as their heterosexual peers, while also enduring higher rates of harassment, discrimination, and violence from within their own units. Discrimination may be overt or take the form of subtle exclusion that undermines unit cohesion; in some cases, they become the "punching bag" of the group.

As a result, LGBTQ+ service members must maintain constant vigilance and live in perpetual fear of discovery, harassment, or violence from the very people who are meant to have their backs. Whether in combat or in their barracks, they are under threat.

Military trauma combined with sexual trauma, harassment, and discrimination means many LGBTQ+ veterans suffer significantly higher rates of PTSD, substance abuse, depressive disorder, anxiety disorders, and suicidal ideation than their heterosexual peers. The military's hypermasculine culture tends to promote homophobia, even though this conflicts with the warrior ethos founded on honor and respect.

To add insult to injury, LGBTQ+ veterans face discrimination from some healthcare providers. As a result, many choose to avoid seeking care.

Psychedelics and LGBTQ+ veterans

For LGBTQ+ service members who were assaulted and harassed in service, a veteran retreat may feel unsafe. We have found that LGBTQ+-specific retreats and integration support give this community a safe space more conducive to recovery. While the military has made strides in addressing MST and harassment, considerable work is yet to be done.

HHP believes that veterans who come together to validate one another's experiences and work toward healing play a crucial role in reform.

BIPOC and undertreated mental health in military service

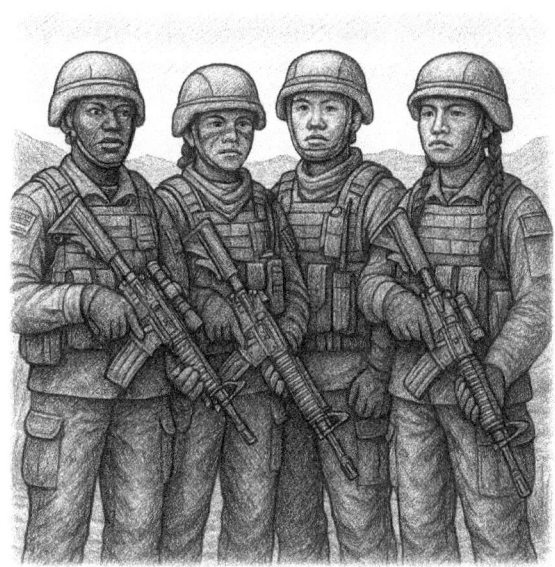

About 40 percent of service members of color report experiencing racial or ethnic discrimination during their service.

While the racial diversity of the U.S. military broadly reflects that of the civilian population, surveys indicate that around 40 percent of service members of color report experiencing racial or ethnic discrimination during their service. As with MST, many fear social or career retaliation if they report these incidents, leading to significant underreporting.

Black Americans have served in every major U.S. conflict since the Revolutionary War, often in segregated units until the armed forces were officially desegregated in 1948. Despite that policy shift, inequities persist, limiting access to leadership roles, elite assignments, and advanced specialties that would lead to faster promotion and post-service career opportunities. Black service members have historically been concentrated in enlisted and combat arms roles and, in conflicts such as Vietnam, suffered disproportionately high casualty rates. Hispanic Americans, who have also served in significant numbers since the nation's founding, have faced similar barriers, including concentration in lower-ranking and high-risk roles. These patterns have likewise affected Native American, Asian American, and Pacific Islander service members.

Discrimination takes many forms, including exclusion, harassment, and violence. Research shows that Black, Indigenous, and other people of color (BIPOC) veterans experience PTSD at significantly higher rates than their white counterparts, with some studies finding prevalence 20–30 percent greater. They also face barriers to care, including cultural stigma within their communities, distrust of medical institutions rooted in historical mistreatment, and difficulty accessing providers who understand both military and racial trauma.

The challenges multiply for BIPOC women in service, who also experience higher rates of sexual harassment and assault than their white female counterparts, and hence higher rates of PTSD and other mental health disorders.

These compounded challenges help explain why BIPOC veterans have higher rates of mental health disorders, including PTSD, depression, anxiety, substance use disorders, and suicidal ideation, than white service members.

Psychedelics in the BIPOC community
White people dominate the psychedelic space, which may feel off-putting to people of color. As with other marginalized veteran communities, HHP works to create BIPOC-specific veteran retreats to allow them to experience psychedelic healing as safely and freely as possible.

——————The Double Battle: Female Veterans——————

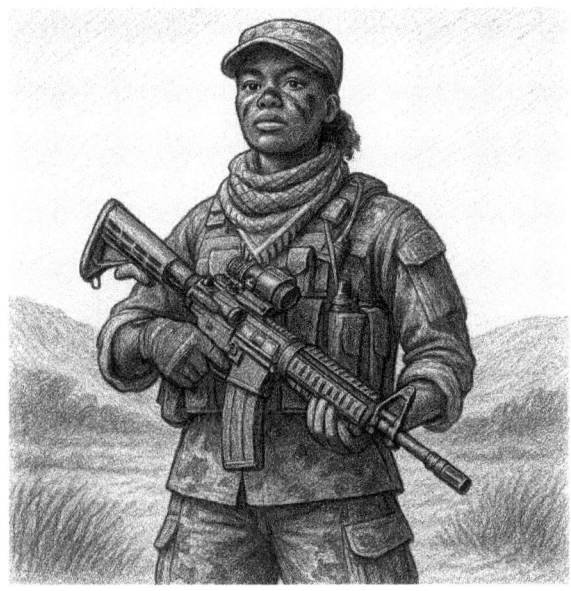

Women have served as warriors throughout history, but face discrimination and MST in modern militaries. The problem is even worse for women of color.

Women have served as warriors throughout history. Archaeological evidence and historical records reveal that women participated in warfare in cultures across the globe, including the Scythians of the Eurasian steppes, the Celtic tribes of Europe, the Viking Age, and the onna-bugeisha in feudal Japan. In the American Revolution, some women disguised themselves as men to fight, while others supported the war effort as spies and nurses. Throughout history, women have played roles in defense, raiding, and survival.

With the rise of industrial-era standing armies, they became more rigidly structured and gender-segregated. As a result, women's contributions were increasingly written out of official histories.

Today's struggle for women's full recognition in the armed forces is not a modern experiment, but a reclamation of a role that women have occupied across many cultures throughout history. Yet women often encounter a military culture that treats them as unwelcome intruders. Many face daily unwanted advances, derogatory comments, hostility from peers, and alarmingly high rates of sexual harassment and assault. Studies estimate that between 55 and 80 percent of servicewomen experience sexual harassment, and around 15–25 percent report military sexual trauma (MST). For some, the threat environment is so constant that they maintain combat readiness even in rest, sometimes even sleeping with firearms.

Service also brings career discrimination: women remain underrepresented in leadership, are passed over for promotions, and are excluded from informal professional networks that advance careers. Once discharged, they face a civilian culture that assumes they are a veteran's spouse rather than the veteran, and even some VA providers question their combat service.

The combination of combat or service-related trauma, sexual trauma, and systemic discrimination is associated with higher rates of PTSD and other mental health challenges among women compared to their male counterparts. More than half of women who experience MST develop PTSD, and studies estimate that 30–40 percent also develop major depressive disorder.

Psychedelics and female veterans
HHP's early retreats brought together female veteran spouses and former members of the Cultural Support Teams, the elite female soldiers who served in combat alongside special operations forces. However, it became clear that female veterans needed a community of peers for psychedelic retreats.

In women-only spaces, female veterans can lower their guard to more effectively explore and process the traumas of military and combat service, discrimination, and MST. Overall, in the general population, more women than men suffer from PTSD, with sexual abuse playing a significant role in that statistic. Female veterans can thrive in women-only spaces to address the traumas they experienced.

CHAPTER 9

PSYCHEDELIC HEALING FOR
VETERAN SPOUSES

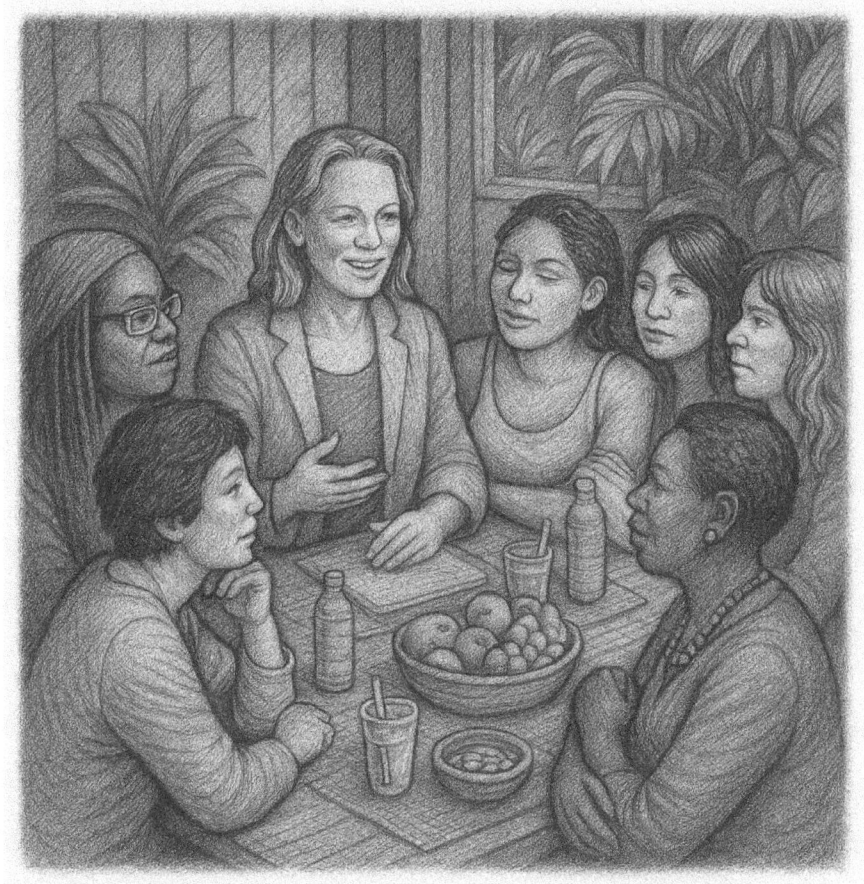

*Veterans' spouses and families may suffer from secondary
PTSD. Veteran spousal healing supports veteran healing.*

Military service is hard on marriages. Veterans experience higher divorce rates compared to civilians, and these rates increase with longer service duration, combat exposure, PTSD development, or involvement in special operations units.

Spouses and partners of veterans can develop what researchers call "secondary PTSD"—distress in response to the trauma of others. Symptoms include anxiety, depression, substance abuse, suicidal ideation, and caregiver fatigue. Children are also affected, leading to the intergenerational transmission of trauma.

In a nutshell, the alienation or PTSD that many discharged service members bring home with them affects the entire family. What's more, failure to address secondary PTSD can thwart the impact of veteran psychedelic therapy. *Spousal healing is integral to veteran healing.*

Veteran Voices

When Allison Wilson's Navy SEAL husband returned from a psychedelic retreat in Mexico, she was anything but supportive. Instead, her husband's retreat ignited her long-smoldering resentment, turning it into rage. At the time, both were steeped in suicidal ideation, depression, a reliance on prescription medications and alcohol to cope, and volatility in their relationship.

"When he went to the psychedelic retreat, I was left at home with five kids and feeling like I didn't have an opportunity to heal," Allison said. "He came home feeling vulnerable and open, and I felt a ball of anger. It caused him to retreat back into a darker space."

Despite her reservations, Wilson eventually went to a psychedelic retreat for veteran spouses. The experience so transformed her that she immediately founded The Hope Project, a non-profit organization that supports veteran spouses.

Many spouses don't feel deserving of healing, or they minimize their experience because they didn't serve, go to war, or develop PTSD. But the reality is that their partner's declining mental health significantly affects their own.

Wilson's husband was deployed up to 300 days a year while she raised their five children alone. She never knew whether he would come home alive; combat death in their community was normalized, and the command occasionally called her with instructions to "hold it together" for her husband. Many spouses feel like they and their children come second to the military.

When a veteran returns from service or combat, they must relearn how to be a civilian, a partner, and a parent, often while battling depression, rage, self-loathing, substance abuse, suicidal ideation, TBI, loss of purpose, or other service "souvenirs."

As a result, many spouses feel they must walk on eggshells around their partner to avoid triggering a meltdown or fit of rage—and also teach their children to do the same. Over time, the constant stress keeps the spouse in a chronic fight-or-flight state while the gap between the couple widens and resentment builds. Some spouses may feel driven to "fix" their partners at the expense of their well-being, or wonder who the stranger is sharing their bed and how they're supposed to reconnect with them.

———Psychedelic healing for spouses and marriages———

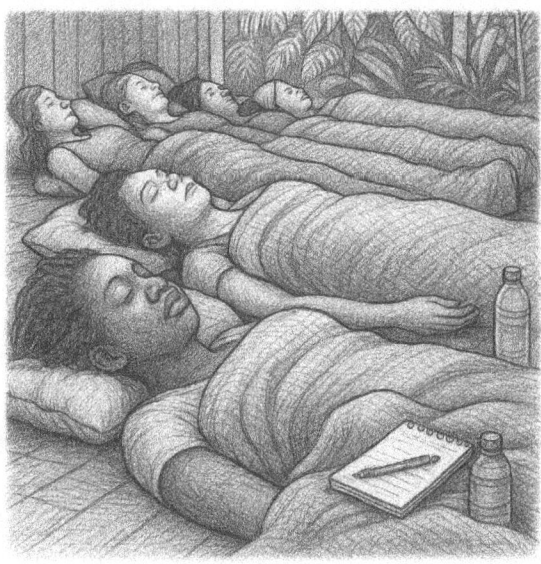

When spouses join retreats with other spouses, it's the first time many realize they aren't alone with their feelings and experiences.

Wilson says successful psychedelic integration depends on a sound support system at home, something she was not emotionally equipped to offer her husband until she found her own support.

"We are all good at zipping up our armor and piling everything down inside of us until we're not. That's when the rage, the drinking, and the suicide happen," she said.

When spouses join retreats with other spouses, it's the first time many realize they aren't alone with their feelings and experiences. Witnessing the same struggles in other spouses and working through the healing journey together opens the door to self-forgiveness and compassion. Having put themselves last for so long, the psychedelic retreats are the first time they can focus on their own well-being without interruption.

The Hope Project has seen most of its participants not only stay in their marriages but also rewrite them. Couples learn new ways to communicate and navigate old patterns with less emotional charge, more openness, and a mutual commitment to their healing.

"The spouses that go through the program have a community they can turn to now," Wilson said. "They now know they can prioritize their well-being, which helps them live from their heart instead of their head."

When healing is a joint venture, partners can "co-regulate," or actively help each other manage their emotional responses, particularly during stress or conflict. Researchers consider this dynamic essential for couples dealing with the aftermath of trauma. Examples of co-regulation include active listening, empathy, and shared coping strategies.

Spousal healing after the death of a veteran
The person who loses a veteran spouse or partner to suicide also loses the opportunity to heal with their partner. Instead, they are left to grieve their partner's death while carrying the burden of secondary PTSD and navigating anger, grief, guilt, and sometimes even relief.

Tambi Lane's partner died by suicide not long after their separation. For years, Lane had to walk on eggshells around him. To friends and family, he was a big, generous softie. But every few months, an unpredictable trigger would send him into an uncontrollable rage. Though he never physically attacked Lane, he punched holes in walls and doors, hurled objects, and terrified everyone around him. Afterward, he would collapse into crushing guilt and shame, numbing himself with alcohol and feeling too unworthy to seek help. Then, life would return to normal until the next trigger set him off.

Lane knew her partner was consumed by remorse over these episodes. She believes undiagnosed autism and TBI acquired as a tank gunner contributed to his mental health burdens.

The couple learned about psilocybin therapy from a documentary and discussed seeking help when Oregon voters approved legal psilocybin services in 2020. But just days before the first service center opened, he took his life. "I had no idea we were on a deadline with his life," Lane said.

Exhausted from years of living with a veteran with PTSD while grieving his death, Lane reached rock bottom. She decided to follow through with their discussion and underwent her first psilocybin journey with a friend who is a facilitator. She credits the experience with helping her process her grief, hold onto positive memories, and release shame, guilt, and fear of judgment.

"Through psilocybin, I was able to spend time with my best friend again, feeling his presence so strongly it brought me to tears," said Lane. "The experience reminded me that love continues beyond death, and that connection is stronger than loss. I could feel how deeply he still cared for me."

Now, Lane is committed to raising awareness so others might find help before it's too late..

CHAPTER 10

PSYCHEDELIC THERAPY FOR FIRST RESPONDERS

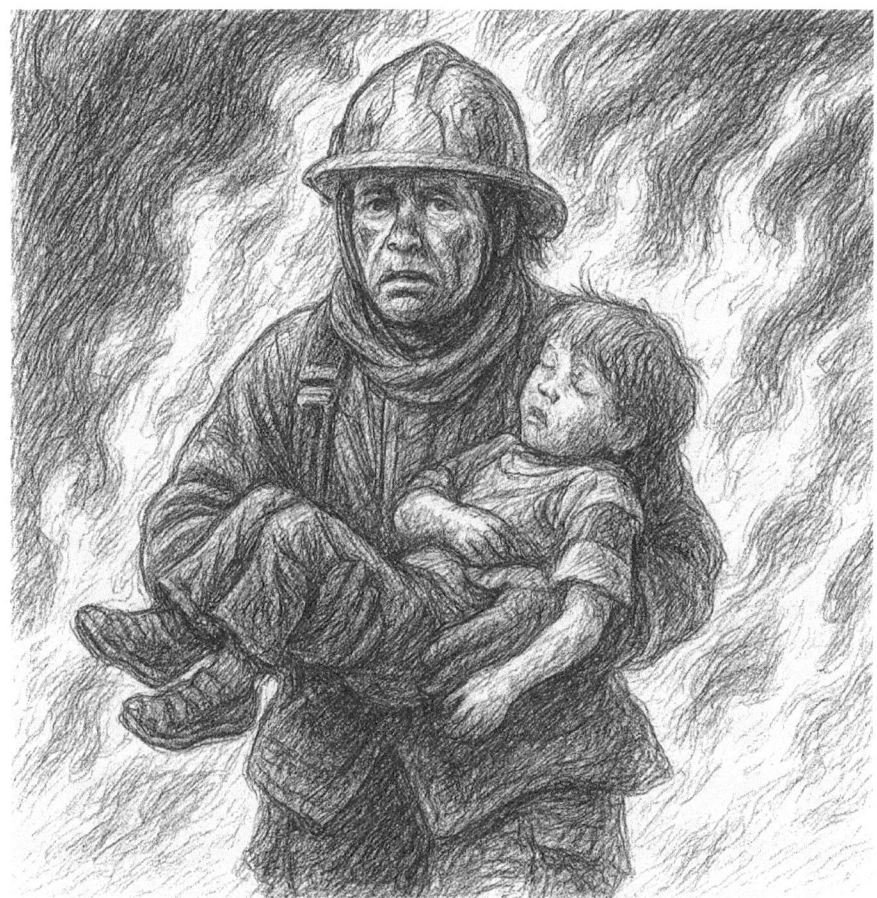

Psychedelic and MDMA therapies help first responders for many of the same reasons they help veterans.

Veterans and first responders share many similarities. Both suffer trauma and PTSD at significantly higher rates than the rest of the population, along with related disorders such as depression, anxiety, suicidal ideation, and substance abuse.

These careers attract those who feel called to serve, often at great personal sacrifice, and they require intense training. Many in both populations already have PTSD from early childhood trauma when entering service. They operate within strict hierarchies that prioritize the collective over the individual. Both groups witness high rates of death, injury, and violence that most civilians rarely encounter. A firefighter who responds to more than 12,000 emergency calls during their career will experience over a hundred traumatic events, whereas the average citizen encounters two to four traumatic events in their lifetime.

The physical toll—sometimes career-ending—and regular exposure to fire-related toxins represent other shared risks. Additionally, both careers become central to personal identity, creating intense social bonds and tight-knit communities that can leave many feeling adrift and isolated after leaving.

"When they no longer carry that title or get to ride around in the big red engine, there's a crisis; they don't know who they are," says Tim Houweling, co-founder with Angela Graham of The S.I.R.E.N. Project, which stands for Supporting Initial Responders with Entheogenic Networking. "They also think that when they retire, now that they're away from the day-to-day calls, those traumas go away. That doesn't happen for a lot of them."

While both careers share similarities, some variations explain why treatment approaches designed for veterans may need adaptation when applied to first responders.

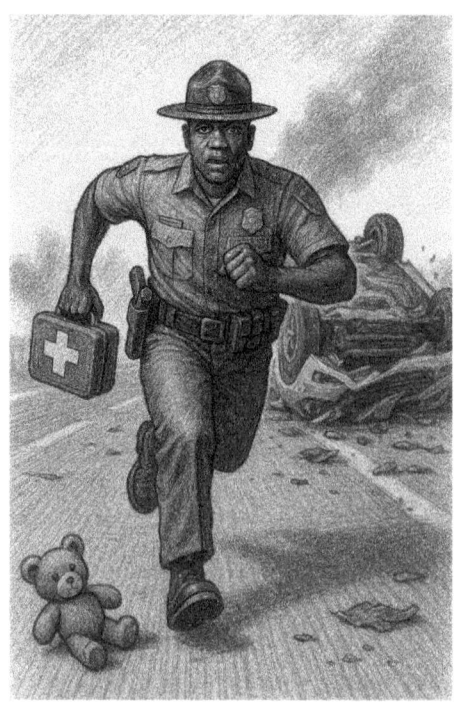

As we've seen, both first responders and veterans experience more traumas on the job compared to civilians. For veterans, this can be through deployment periods, training accidents, or violence or harassment from within their teams during careers that average four to eight years. However, first responders face trauma exposure regularly over a career of 25 to 30 years, sometimes having to drive past the location of a particularly traumatic event daily.

First responders may have to drive past the location of a particularly traumatic experience on a daily basis.

Further, although soldiers often serve in reactive situations, such as during patrols or peacekeeping duties, their roles tend to be more proactive and mission-oriented, which involves psychological and tactical preparation. First responders typically respond to emergencies that occur in day-to-day life, creating an atmosphere of chronic unpredictability that can heighten stress responses.

It is significant that first-responder careers are typically lifelong, and engaging in psychedelic therapy can jeopardize their job.

Because psychedelics are given the same federal classification as deadly and addictive drugs like fentanyl and methamphetamine, first responders face the moral complexity of enforcing drug laws while seeking psychedelic healing.

The worsening mental health crisis among first responders

The first responder mental health crisis has intensified over the past two decades, with firefighter suicide rates having increased by approximately 500 percent since 2000. Divorce rates among firefighters reach up to 80 percent in some departments.

Because first responders become so adept at dissociation to respond to emergency situations, standard therapies frequently fail to break through these protective barriers.

Stigmas around mental health and fears about job security can discourage first responders from seeking help before they reach a crisis. Department policies make this worse by requiring officers to report mental health issues and offering little confidentiality. This fosters a "push it down" mentality.

The consequences of this avoidance can hit like a wrecking ball upon retirement. Suddenly, they lose their community and sense of identity, and the decades of suppressed trauma come rushing to the surface. This combination creates what Houweling describes as "the recipe for suicide:" a mix of isolation from a protective community, loss of purposeful identity, often chronic pain, and decades of unprocessed trauma suddenly surfacing without the distractions of daily emergency response.

Psychedelic therapy for first responders who are still actively employed

Unlike veterans, who typically seek treatment post-service, first responders must navigate ongoing sleep deprivation, constantly shifting schedules, and an immediate return to potentially traumatic work environments following their psychedelic journeys, all while risking career termination under current drug laws.

The S.I.R.E.N. Project is one organization that has emerged to address mental health issues in the first responder community by hosting retreats in Mexico, where psychedelic ceremonies are legal. This allows participants to state truthfully that they've never violated U.S. law. Their integration practices focus on building resilience in the face of ongoing trauma exposure, rather than simply processing past experiences. Their community-based healing emphasizes confidentiality and career protection.

Despite the challenges, Houweling sees the culture shifting as more personnel experience the benefits of psychedelic therapy. In his own department, where approximately 20 percent of staff have participated in psychedelic therapy, the changes are visible. "There are guys who are in their station doing Wim Hof breathing, meditating openly. That would never, ever have happened even five years ago," he says.

This grassroots approach is proving more effective than top-down policy changes, as it shifts the culture through word of mouth while helping first responders.

How psychedelic therapy is changing mental health outcomes among first responders

While formal research remains limited, first responders who have participated in psychedelic therapy often report reductions in intrusive memories, improved sleep quality, decreased hypervigilance, heightened compassion and empathy, and diminished reliance on alcohol and medications. Many describe a newfound mental clarity and relief from emotional burden.

Despite these promising observations, no large-scale, first-responder-specific outcome studies have been conducted. Creating anonymous reporting structures for tracking long-term outcomes, particularly after retirement, would provide valuable data for improving interventions.

"My healing journey made me think of all my friends and family who have been suffering or have died by suicide, and how this could have saved them," S.I.R.E.N. cofounder Angela Graham says. "I sought help for my PTSD after 20 years of experience because I was so far gone. You wanna discipline me for that? I will take that fight every day of the week."

CHAPTER 11

A NEEDED PARADIGM SHIFT
IN HEALTHCARE BELIEFS

While modern medicine is miraculous in acute and life-or-death situations, the standard healthcare model is failing in the mental health and suicide crisis among veterans.

One of the biggest hurdles we encounter in veterans, policymakers, and the culture at large is the belief in the "pill for a symptom" model of health. This paradigm is why many veterans end up on up to a dozen different psychiatric medications. These medications often come with side effects, diminishing returns over time, and debilitating dependency.

The psychedelic therapy paradigm recognizes symptoms as warning signs of deeper problems and seeks to address the root cause of those problems, rather than masking them with medications. At HHP, we are not anti-medication but rather pro-genuine healing.

Five foundations of the
psychedelic healing paradigm

Psychedelic therapy challenges everything we've been taught about mental health treatment. Unlike traditional approaches that focus on medicating symptoms, psychedelic healing demands active participation in one's own recovery.

This paradigm shift isn't easy. It asks one to question deeply held beliefs about medication, quick fixes, and surface-level solutions, and instead requires them to investigate the root causes. Most importantly, it requires a commitment to a comprehensive overhaul of one's mindset and lifestyle.

The following five foundations represent core principles of psychedelic healing, and a reimagining of what veteran healing can look like. While they may seem initially demanding, they reflect what research and veteran experiences have shown: lasting healing requires veterans to transcend from passive patients into active architects of their own evolution.

Five foundations of psychedelic healing:

1. Self-curiosity: Willingness to explore internally

2. Rejecting false and outdated thinking: Dismiss the propaganda about psychedelics

3. Personalized care: No one-size-fits-all solutions

4. Embracing preparation and integration: Honoring the entire healing process

5. Implementing a brain-healthy diet and lifestyle: Giving the brain the right environment to heal

---

1. Self-curiosity

Psychedelic therapy is rarely a "one-and-done" path to recovery. It requires a willingness to look deeply under the hood of one's own mind, uncover the toxic sources of dysfunction, and fully immerse oneself in the difficult work of recovery.

Occasionally, a psychedelic experience is so profound that a veteran emerges feeling "healed." More often, however, psychedelics disrupt the brain's default patterns long enough for the veteran to step outside entrenched neurological ruts. This creates a window of opportunity to break free from cycles of avoidance and suppression, confront trauma without falling apart, and reframe life through a more positive and constructive lens.

This approach is about understanding and integrating pain, not masking it.

2. Rejecting false and outdated thinking

This paradigm shift requires one to reject the stigma surrounding psychedelics and instead turn toward decades of scientific data and tens of thousands of positive anecdotes. Although psychedelics are not appropriate for everyone, when used responsibly and in a therapeutic context, they can be powerful tools for healing.

3. Personalized care

The psychedelic paradigm shift recognizes that healing is not a one-size-fits-all process. It calls for a personalized approach that accounts for each person's unique experiences, needs, and goals. Ten different people with combat or service trauma may require ten different healing pathways tailored to their unique backgrounds, personalities, and ways of living.

4. Embracing preparation and integration

The psychedelic paradigm honors the entire healing process, not just the journey itself. Preparation and integration are given as much, if not more, importance than the psychedelic experience. Integration can involve processing overwhelming emotions, rebuilding trust, and discovering new meaning and purpose. This process is strengthened by the support of therapists, peers, and a veteran community, creating a network that sustains healing long after the session ends.

5. Implementing a brain-healthy diet and lifestyle

Psychedelic therapy works best if the brain's environment is not compromised by a sedentary lifestyle, junk foods, substance abuse, stressful relationships, and other factors that undermine brain health. Psychedelic healing is best supported through brain-healthy practices such as regular exercise, positive social interaction, healthy eating, and the avoidance of numbing substances that promote depression and anxiety.

———Conclusion———

For psychedelic therapy to exert its maximum potential, we must shift cultural and institutional paradigms to address the root causes of mental health disorders. This ensures lasting and sustainable improvement versus a medication model that masks symptoms and fosters drug dependence.

CHAPTER 12

COMMON PSYCHEDELICS FOR MENTAL HEALTH RECOVERY

At this point, we still don't have enough evidence to determine which psychedelic is best suited for a given individual or set of circumstances. However, after nearly a decade of connecting veterans with psychedelic services, clear patterns have emerged that distinguish the different types of psychedelic experiences.

As of 2025, the main psychedelics being used for veterans are psilocybin, ayahuasca, ibogaine, and 5-MeO-DMT.

Though not technically psychedelics, MDMA and ketamine are used in therapeutic and clinical settings, and their federal legal status can make them more accessible. The research on MDMA-assisted therapy for veteran PTSD has opened the doors to the world of psychedelics and helped legitimize their therapeutic use.

People can have the best or the worst of experiences with any psychedelic. However, users report similar experiences, unique to each one.

———Psilocybin, "magic mushrooms"———

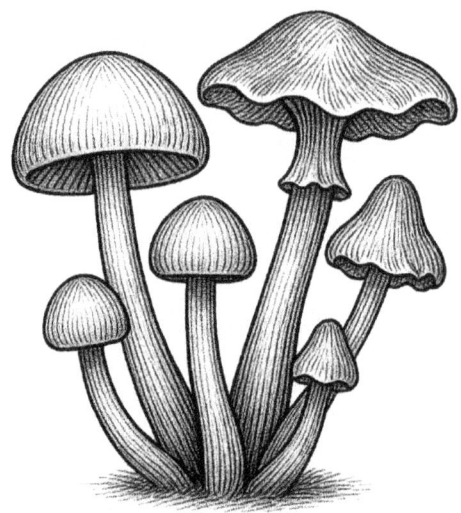

Psilocybin has been studied for conditions such as cluster headaches, obsessive-compulsive disorders, anxiety, depression, PTSD, addiction, and brain injury.

Psilocybin (4-phosphoryloxy-N, N-dimethyltryptamine) made military history in 2023 when Heroic Hearts Project hosted the first legal psychedelic retreat for veterans on American soil. The retreat happened in Bend, Oregon, at one of the country's first legal psilocybin service centers.

Psilocybin mushrooms are popularly known as "magic mushrooms." They grow naturally in damp areas in decaying organic matter and are popular home-grown projects among amateur mycologists.

Historically, indigenous peoples in Central and South America, Africa, Europe, Siberia, and Southeast Asia have used them. The Aztecs call them *teonanacatl*, meaning "flesh of the gods."

A central figure in the legacy of psilocybin is Maria Sabina, a Mazatec curandera (healer) from Mexico. In the 1950s, American amateur mycologist R. Gordon Wasson introduced her to the West in a *Life* magazine article. While her emphasis on the spiritual properties of psilocybin profoundly impacted the counterculture movement of the '60s and '70s, it also flooded her village with careless tourists who exploited the locals' ancient sacred practices. As a result, her community expelled her in 1962, thrusting her into poverty and regret. Sabina's story is an enduring reminder of the sensitivity required when using indigenous medicines.

More than 180 species of mushrooms contain psilocybin, although the most commonly used is *Psilocybe cubensis*. Popular strains within that species, and their purported qualities, include:

- Golden Teacher: More of a mental than a visual experience.
- B+ (Be Positive): An all-purpose psilocybin experience.
- Penis Envy: Known for its potency and its distinct shape.
- Liberty Caps: Grows wild worldwide; known for a more visual experience.

While psilocybin has its roots in indigenous spiritual practices worldwide, research demonstrates its multiple therapeutic benefits. It has been studied for conditions such as cluster headaches, obsessive-compulsive disorders, anxiety, depression, PTSD, addiction, and brain injury.

The psilocybin experience
Psilocybin is a psychedelic staple for newcomers and experienced journeyers alike. Users typically ingest psilocybin mushrooms dried, but they can also be consumed as tea, in chocolate, or in capsules.

Potency can vary depending on the strain and even the batch.

Psilocybin is perhaps the most popular compound used for microdosing at 0.1–0.3g doses. The user does not experience an altered state with microdosing, but many report improved mood and energy on a microdosing regimen.

From there, doses and effects can range from mild to massive. Typical doses for a psychedelic journey start in the range of 2–3.5g, with "heroic" doses going from 5g and up.

The effects typically begin within twenty to forty minutes of ingestion, with the peak experience occurring around two to three hours after ingestion. The journey can last 4 to 6 hours, and the effects linger for several more hours.

How psilocybin differs from other psychedelics
Compared to ayahuasca or ibogaine, the psilocybin experience is often described as grounding, earthy, and playful. We refer to it as the general practitioner, whereas the others are specialists or surgeons.

Psilocybin offers a well-rounded introduction to the psychedelic experience. Compared to other psychedelics, it tends to provide a gentler user entry.

However, don't be complacent; a large dose or a potent strain can thrust one into a powerful hallucinogenic experience.

In veteran mental health support, psilocybin is used in a ceremonial group or individual setting under the guidance of trained facilitators. Journeys last five or six hours. It is generally safe and does not require medical supervision like ibogaine or ketamine. An added benefit of psilocybin is that it is safe and effective for those taking SSRIs, although a higher dose is typically needed.

HHP typically schedules psilocybin journeys over two to three nights. For the newcomer, the first night can introduce the "shock value" of the psychedelic experience and unearth buried inner material. A mild tolerance develops on subsequent nights, and the user may need larger doses for a deeper dive after the initial relationship with the medicine has been established. This differs from ayahuasca, with which the experiences can grow in power over subsequent nights. Psilocybin helps many veterans with a much-needed neurological reset. Users report greater self-understanding after their experiences.

Psilocybin for veteran PTSD

Psilocybin is used in group and individual settings to address veteran PTSD and mental health issues. The compound has largely been studied to support depression and cancer-related anxiety, but its role in addressing PTSD and brain injury are being investigated.

In 2019, the FDA designated psilocybin therapy as a "breakthrough therapy" for depression, fast-tracking its review and development, a status that has since been extended to new psilocybin-based compounds.

————Ketamine, "the K-hole"————

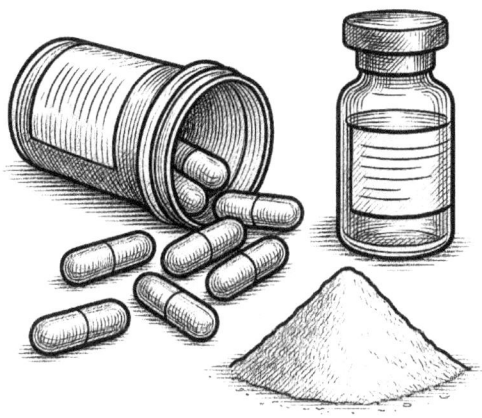

Many ketamine users report dramatic and swift relief from depression, suicidality, and PTSD in a series of sessions in clinical ketamine settings. Studies also suggest it can support healing from traumatic brain injury (TBI).

Ketamine ((RS)-2-(2-Chlorophenyl)-2-(methylamino)cyclohexanone) is a psychedelic outlier as it's technically an anesthetic, but it can provide immediate relief for suicidality and severe depression. It also has the bonus of being federally legal, with both in-person and online ketamine clinics existing around the country.

Some contend that ketamine's therapeutic use for mental health originated on the battlefront. A 2008 study showed soldiers burned in battle who received ketamine had a lower prevalence rate of PTSD later compared to those who had not, despite higher injuries, more surgeries, and more time in intensive care. While a follow-up study six years later disputed this finding, ketamine has nevertheless proven a valuable tool in managing PTSD, depression, and other mental health issues veterans face.

The ketamine experience
Ketamine is a dissociative anesthetic that induces a sense of detachment from the body and profound changes in perception. Many users report dramatic and swift relief from depression, suicidality, and PTSD in a series of sessions in clinical settings. Studies also suggest it can support healing from TBI.

Most ketamine clinics offer ketamine in an intravenous infusion or intra-muscular injection. A Zoom session may involve the patient using ketamine lozenges at home while working with the facilitator online. Patients may also be prescribed ketamine sublingual lozenges or nasal spray in lower dosages to use more regularly between infusions.

An intense ketamine experience is referred to as the "K-hole" in club slang.

The current ketamine controversy
While Rketamine (arketamine) remains the most commonly used form of ketamine for depression and suicidality, such use is off-label. It is widely and legally administered as a generic, with its popularity stemming from its accessibility rather than regulatory approval.

That began shifting in 2019 with the FDA's approval of Spravato, a branded Sketamine (esketamine) nasal spray indicated for treatment-resistant depression. S-ketamine shares many effects with R-ketamine but benefits from FDA approval, which means it's insurance-covered (with some caveats) and significantly more expensive.

Recent clinical findings suggest that intravenous racemic ketamine (a mix of both R- and Sketamine) may provide stronger antidepressant responses and higher remission rates than S-ketamine, though head-to-head trials are still ongoing.

At the same time, Spravato's FDA approval has been expanded to allow its use as a monotherapy (meaning they no longer require therapy to be accompanied by oral antidepressants), increasing its accessibility and flexibility in treatment.

In real-world and research settings, ketamine (in its various forms) continues to demonstrate rapid reductions in suicidal ideation, making it invaluable during mental health crises. However, its effects may be short-lived.

Ultimately, deciding between R-ketamine, racemic ketamine, or S-ketamine will depend on availability, affordability, and clinical context.

How ketamine differs from other psychedelics
With music and therapeutic guidance, ketamine can put the user into a psychedelic-like experience. People report "melting" into a detached state, allowing them to gain a zoomed-out perspective on themselves and their issues. Many also report feelings of self-love and compassion from this new vantage point.

A therapist can optimize that state by guiding the participant into areas of unresolved trauma and mental blockages. Undergoing treatment in a clinical setting with a veteran-trained therapist is preferable to the at-home Zoom model if there is tension or conflict in the home environment.

Because it helps many people experience immediate relief from severe depression and suicidality, it can be an effective intervention in crisis situations.

Ketamine also differs from other psychedelics in other ways:

Ketamine differs from other psychedelics in several ways:

1. It's legal.
2. It has the potential to be habit-forming.
3. Its results are possibly only temporary.
4. It can have health risks.

It's legal

Ketamine is legally accessible. The FDA has approved R-ketamine for "off-label" use for depression, PTSD, suicidality, chronic pain, and other disorders. Infusion therapy clinics have popped up around the country, online clinics offer ketamine sessions via Zoom, and some people use ketamine lozenges or a nasal spray daily to keep symptoms at bay.

S-ketamine, under the brand label Spravato, is FDA-approved for treatment-resistant depression.

It has the potential to be habit-forming

Some people develop a dependency on ketamine. It's unusual for psychedelics to become habit-forming; however, ketamine is a popular club drug that many people abuse. If you are prone to substance use disorder, it's suggested you avoid ketamine.

Its results are possibly only temporary

Ketamine results are not necessarily long-lasting. Most psychedelics support healing through breakthrough mystical experiences that help rewire the brain so that dependence is not required.

Ketamine therapy, on the other hand, often requires repeat visits every six weeks or so to keep symptoms at bay. However, studies show it reduces symptoms of PTSD, and many users also report breakthrough experiences on ketamine that, with integration support, help them work through their issues and alleviate symptoms.

It can have health risks

Ketamine is relatively safe and non-toxic for prescribed therapeutic use. However, habitual users may experience cognitive impairment and bladder pain or damage.

Ketamine for veteran PTSD

Two of ketamine's most significant selling points are that it's easier to access in the U.S. than other psychedelics and that its antidepressant and anti-anxiety effects can be immediate. For the veteran struggling with severe suicidality, this can be lifesaving. It has also been shown to help reduce symptoms of PTSD (though results are mixed), support mood regulation, and promote healing from brain injury.

Veteran Voices

Army medic veteran Carl Bonnett, MD, has a background in emergency medicine and now works with veterans using ketamine therapy. He recalled the poignant turnaround he witnessed in a veteran who had served as a sniper.

"He saw some horrible black ops stuff that would not play well on CNN," Bonnett said. "His whole job was to hunt and kill human beings. There is a thin line between the civilized man and the savage. He was thinking about some of the things he had done, then looking at his own kids. The ketamine helped him detach and start to remodel who he was as a person.

"It took him about three years to finally start getting into a good space. Now, he's working for a nonprofit, and he's not an angry person anymore.

"It takes a tremendous amount of reprogramming, especially with someone like him, who is a special operations sniper.

"The ketamine helps get people through the door, but then they must start doing the work. There is a lot of personal work and growth that needs to be done."

———LSD, "acid"———

Before the "War on Drugs" legislative campaign of the late twentieth century, LSD was on its way to becoming a psychiatric tool for depression and other mental health disorders, with thousands of people already undergoing treatment.

LSD (lysergic acid diethylamide) is perhaps the most embedded psychedelic in the cultural consciousness, thanks to the hippie movement of the '60s and '70s and the subsequent psychedelic smear campaign that persists today.

Swiss scientist Albert Hoffman discovered LSD in 1938. However, when Timothy Leary and Richard Alpert (Ram Dass)'s research on its therapeutic use at Harvard University leaked into the counterculture, it became synonymous with the anti-war hippie movement, eventually leading to Leary's and Alpert's dismissal from Harvard.

During the same period, military and intelligence agencies conducted a series of experiments to assess LSD's potential applications for mind control, interrogation, and behavior modification. The experiments ultimately showed the nature of LSD to be chaotic and unpredictable, with military test subjects often succumbing to fits of laughter.

The Silicon Valley tech boom has its roots in the early days of LSD, with trailblazers like Steve Jobs crediting their visionary innovations in part to LSD. LSD's role in Silicon Valley again flourished in the 2010s when microdosing (regularly taking doses too small to be psychoactive) became a popular way to boost creativity and productivity.

Another historical side note about LSD is its role in Alcoholics Anonymous. Bill Wilson, co-founder of AA, experimented with LSD in the 1950s. He believed that the spiritual awakening and shifts in consciousness many experienced with LSD could help people overcome alcohol addiction.

The LSD experience

LSD is less commonly used in group retreats or individual facilitation sessions, possibly due to its duration. An LSD trip can last twelve hours or more.

LSD is typically consumed on blotter paper, in liquid form, or in a gel tab. The effects can begin as little as thirty minutes after ingestion, with the peak experience kicking in four to six hours later.

LSD is commonly used for microdosing by diluting a dose in a small container with distilled water.

How LSD differs from other psychedelics

HHP has generally avoided LSD from an advocacy standpoint due to its political "baggage." It still carries significant stigma from the '60s and '70s, and merely mentioning it can shut down conversations with curious lawmakers or potential donors.

Because it lasts a long time and is synthetic, requiring reputable sourcing, it presents too many barriers to widespread adoption by the veteran community.

LSD for veteran PTSD

Before President Nixon's "War on Drugs" quashed psychedelic research, LSD was on its way to becoming a psychiatric tool for depression and other mental health disorders, with thousands of people already undergoing treatment. More than 1,000 academic papers and books were published on the therapeutic use of LSD. More recent studies have shown that LSD is effective in alleviating end-of-life anxiety, life-threatening illness anxiety, and alcoholism. There is scant research on its application for PTSD.

———Ayahuasca, "grandmother medicine" ———

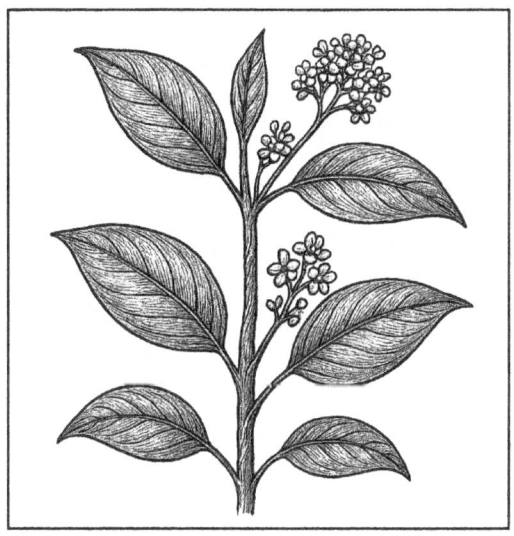

Ayahuasca retreats are a mainstay in the veteran psychedelic community, both in underground circles in the United States and at legal retreat centers in Central and South America. Anecdotal reports about the medicine's therapeutic potential for PTSD are abundant.

Ayahuasca is referred to as "grandmother medicine," and after a few journeys, it's clear why: she can give you unprecedented care and compassion one night and a well-deserved spanking the next.

Ayahuasca is made by brewing *Banisteriopsis caapi* leaves containing DMT, a powerful psychoactive substance, with a vine that inhibits the enzyme that breaks down DMT in the gut. Its history dates back centuries among the people of the Amazon, where it is revered as the mother of all plant medicines. In the Quechuan language, its name means "vine of the soul."

A shaman, or *curandero* (medicine person), guides a traditional ayahuasca journey in the Amazon. Facilitators trained in these practices guide group ceremonies in the West. While shamans are sought for their healing support these days, traditionally, they drank ayahuasca to access the spirit realms and divine information about planting, harvesting, hunting, community issues, sickness, and warfare.

The ayahuasca experience

The ayahuasca experience typically takes place in a group led by a shaman or facilitator, with the aid of one or more helpers. Participants are asked to prepare for two to four weeks before the ceremony by following a "dieta"—a strict diet and abstention from alcohol, caffeine, cannabis, and other mind-altering substances. Several days prior, it's essential to avoid foods high in tyramines, a compound that can interact with the MAO inhibitors in the brew. These foods include aged cheeses, cured or smoked meats, fermented foods, and alcoholic beverages.

During the journey, each person consumes a small cup of the ayahuasca brew one to two times. Music figures prominently into the evening, including *Icaros*, traditional songs integral to the indigenous shamanic practices of the Amazon.

The effects begin thirty to sixty minutes after ingestion, peak in two to four hours, and last six to eight hours.

The ayahuasca experience can be profound, offering piercing insights, revelations, and valuable lessons.

For some, the experience is very visual, with multi-colored fractals and geometric patterns. They often report visions of jungle animals and plants, ancient times and places, aliens and other worlds, and visits from loved ones who have died.

Ayahuasca also immerses the user into recesses of the psyche, areas that have long been suppressed but that may underlie mental health issues. The first few ceremonies plunge some users into long-suppressed underworlds of isolation, grief, and despair. After one or more of these visceral, somatic immersions into unresolved darkness, many veterans report that they eventually stop fighting the experience and instead submit to it.

This surrender allows them to break into the light of universal oneness and unconditional love. Finding their way out is one way that veterans find a lasting therapeutic effect and neurological reconditioning through ayahuasca. They can see what they have been putting themselves through mentally and physically in terms of self-hate, shame, and guilt, and begin to exercise compassion and self-care instead.

Ayahuasca is served in a group setting over multiple nights, and a narrative arc typically plays out over the course of these nights. The retreat begins with the introductory experience, builds up and crescendos, and then softens and concludes. Most people are able to work through specific themes in this arc.

Ayahuasca can also produce a more physical experience compared to other psychedelics, and vomiting is a common way to "purge" during a ceremony.

Care must be taken with ayahuasca to avoid pharmaceutical contraindications and even certain foods. The user must not be taking SSRIs due to the risk of serotonin syndrome and must avoid cured and fermented foods for several days before the ceremony due to the presence of tyramine in these foods. Tyramine can interact dangerously with MAOIs like ayahuasca, increasing the risk of high blood pressure.

Ayahuasca for veteran PTSD

Ayahuasca retreats are a mainstay in the veteran psychedelic community, both in underground circles in the United States and at legal retreat centers in Central and South America. Although anecdotal reports about the medicine's therapeutic potential for PTSD are abundant, little research has been conducted.

Recently, however, a pilot study involving eight combat veterans found that seven experienced clinically significant improvements in PTSD symptoms, five of whom maintained those gains three months post-treatment (Hearn et al., 2023). A 2025 observational study of veterans attending legal psilocybin or ayahuasca retreats reported sustained improvements across PTSD, depression, anxiety, sleep, and reintegration outcomes, even one month post-retreat (Calnan et al., 2025).

Veteran Voices
Daniel

Before attending his first three-night ayahuasca retreat, Navy veteran Daniel* hoped to understand why rage and anger constantly hijacked him. His first ayahuasca journey immersed him in the memories and trauma of childhood sexual abuse by an older male relative.

"The next morning, I woke up with scrapes on my knees, the tops of my feet, and my elbows," Daniel said. "I had a big bruise on my head. People said it looked like I was fighting a ghost. All that childhood aggression came out."

Jamie

Jamie Fremgen, a Cultural Support Team combat veteran, participated in a Heroic Hearts Project Ayahuasca retreat in Peru. "The experience broke me open," she said. "I went in with the intention of getting in touch with my vulnerability, emotions, and femininity, which I had suppressed for so many

---

*Not his real name.

years to fit in in the military. Ayahuasca needed to break through a lot of layers. I let go of so much anger. When I decided to stop suffering, it was just so beautiful. Ayahuasca taught me that I needed a community and to stop isolating myself. It took my control, but it also introduced me to vulnerability and emotions."

———Ibogaine, "the life review"———

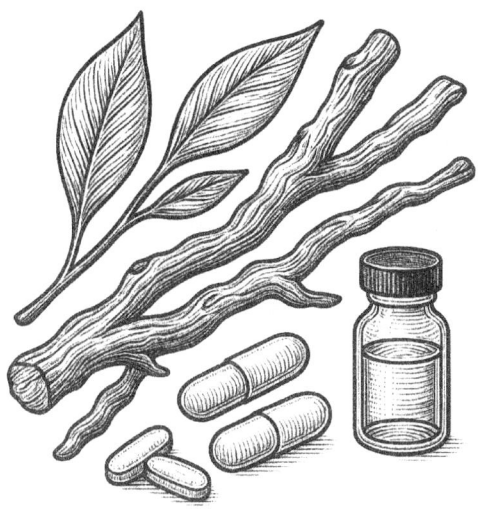

Ibogaine has been shown to ease withdrawal symptoms from heroin, cocaine, and methamphetamine. It has also been shown to support brain healing in special ops vets with traumatic brain injury.

Ibogaine (12-Methoxyibogamine) is best known for treating opiate and other drug addictions. In the veteran psychedelic community, especially at legal retreat centers in Central America, it's also widely used to help process PTSD. A 2024 Stanford-led observational study of Special Operations veterans with traumatic brain injury found that ibogaine, administered with magnesium, produced significant improvements in functioning, PTSD, depression, and anxiety, with no serious adverse events (Cherian et al., 2024). In 2025, Texas committed $50 million in public funding to support clinical trials investigating ibogaine's therapeutic potential for PTSD and addiction, marking a major step toward legitimizing this treatment in the U.S. (Texas Health funding, 2025).

One of the most common reports from the ibogaine experience is a dissociative "life review" unfolding like a slideshow that is uncompromising but benevolent.

Ibogaine is a psychoactive compound derived from the *Tabernanthe iboga* plant found in the rainforests of Central Africa. It is traditionally used for medicinal and ceremonial purposes within the Bwiti religion among the Fang people. It is believed to facilitate communication with ancestors, spirits, and divine entities, which iboga shamans use to help guide community matters and address illnesses.

The CIA studied the effects of ibogaine in the 1950s for its potential use as a "truth serum" in mind control, interrogation techniques, and behavioral manipulation.

The ibogaine experience

Many veterans describe their ibogaine experience as a slideshow that reviews their lives, including the good, the bad, and the ugly. One former Navy SEAL said he was taken through the experience of every person he killed and every death he witnessed in combat, feeling each victim's fear and pain, and hearing, smelling, and sensing everything about the experience in full detail. Yet people report reliving these experiences with a sense of emotional detachment that allows them to process and make peace with them, alleviating the trauma.

While most report challenging but healing journeys, others are shown positive life experiences to remind them that things are not as bad as they think.

The ibogaine experience lasts about twenty-four hours. Users commonly experience difficulty with muscle coordination, dizziness, nausea, vomiting, heartbeat irregularities, and irregular breathing.

Users can expect to lie down for the first twelve hours. The acute phase begins one to three hours after taking ibogaine and can last four to eight hours. This is when the panoramic life review typically occurs. A reflective, evaluative phase of eight to twenty hours follows. The psychoactive effects diminish after twelve to twenty-four hours, and people often report heightened arousal and vigilance. Some report a reduced need for sleep for several days to weeks following treatment.

Ibogaine risks

Ibogaine is unique compared to other psychedelics in that it carries some heart risks. A pre-existing heart condition or specific drug interactions can make ibogaine lethal. Some people suffer a fatal reaction to ibogaine even after a medical screening. It's estimated that up to 1 in 400 people who take ibogaine suffer a deadly reaction.

Therefore, ibogaine should only be taken under the direct supervision of a trained medical professional.

How ibogaine differs from other psychedelics

The ibogaine experience tends to be much more analytical than other psychedelic journeys. Many report seeing their life replayed as a slideshow, on television screens, or in other linear displays. It can be very methodical, allowing the user to connect the dots between specific experiences, behaviors, emotions, or issues.

Because it can cause cardiovascular problems in vulnerable people, people must undergo a medical screening and be medically supervised during the ibogaine experience. The experience lasts about twenty-four hours, and it's very difficult for people to move during this time. People report feeling weighed down, and movement causes nausea.

Ibogaine for veteran PTSD

Case studies and research demonstrate that ibogaine eases withdrawal symptoms for heroin, cocaine, and methamphetamine addicts. A single ibogaine treatment can help relieve cravings for months afterward.

As mentioned, a 2024 study found ibogaine supported brain healing in special ops vets with traumatic brain injuries. Like other psychedelics, ibogaine can also help alleviate PTSD, depression, and anxiety through a powerful mystical experience.

————MDMA, "molly" or "ecstasy"————

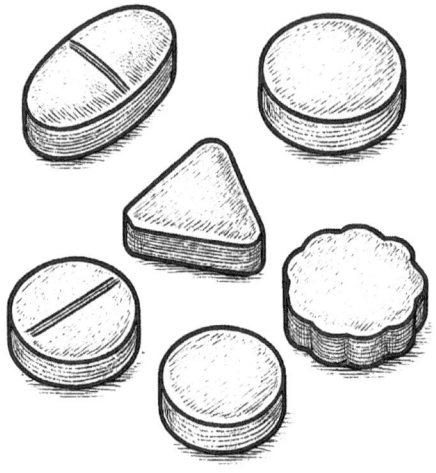

A staggering 71 percent of participants no longer qualified for a PTSD diagnosis after three eight-hour MDMA-assisted therapy sessions. Up to 87 percent experienced clinically significant improvement in their symptoms.

In a therapeutic setting, MDMA (3,4-methylenedioxy-N-methylamphetamine) acts like a psychic scalpel, surgically excising buried trauma while "anesthetizing" the brain's pathways for fear and anger. This allows the participant to process traumatic experiences without triggering a fight-or-flight reaction. Most participants find significant relief from PTSD after their sessions, often describing them as "years of talk therapy condensed into a few hours."

Psychologist and psychotherapist Leo Zeff popularized MDMA in the 1970s to treat depression, calling it "penicillin for the soul." It became reclassified as a Schedule I narcotic in 1985 due to its popularity as a club drug.

Although it's not technically a psychedelic, MDMA has, to date, been the most studied compound for veteran PTSD and has helped pave the way for broader psychedelic research. This is thanks to the trailblazing work of Rick Doblin, the founder of the Multidisciplinary Association for Psychedelic Studies (MAPS). Doblin raised private funding and launched a pilot study on veterans in 2010 with dramatic results and ongoing clinical trials.

In 2023, Congress approved $20 million for the VA to begin MDMA-assisted therapies for veterans starting in 2025.

The MDMA-assisted therapy experience
MDMA is a much different experience in a therapeutic setting than at a club or festival.

In clinical trials, doses of MDMA range between 80 and 150mg. Effects begin in about twenty to sixty minutes, and the experience lasts three to five hours.

Typical effects include euphoria, emotional openness, emotional security, and reduced inhibitions. Connecting with others becomes easy, allowing the participant to bond with the therapist while plunging into an inner journey. This connection is believed to be the "secret sauce" in MDMA's healing potential compared to doing the drug alone or in a recreational setting.

These effects also make MDMA a powerful tool in couples therapy, allowing couples to work through issues without being triggered.

MDMA risks
Adverse effects of MDMA may include elevated blood pressure and heart rate, tremors, jaw clenching, urinary urgency, hot and cold flushes, and insomnia. MDMA overdoses can be lethal.

Because MDMA acts on serotonin pathways, users commonly report fatigue and depression after use. Some say taking 5-HTP or tryptophan before MDMA-assisted therapy may help prevent depression after the experience.

However, research suggests participants in clinical trials experience an MDMA "afterglow" rather than depression because they are given pure MDMA instead of adulterated street MDMA.

MDMA in the veteran psychedelic landscape
Although MDMA has been grouped with psychedelics, it's more of a psychedelic cousin in a traditional talk therapy setting. Under the influence of MDMA, the veteran can let down long-held walls, experience trust and vulnerability, and bond with the therapist. This allows one to dive into buried traumas to unearth and process them.

Whereas most psychedelics transport one to alternate realms to process trauma, MDMA offers a straightforward and literal connection. The ability to talk through traumas without triggering fear and anxiety helps make future therapy sessions more open and productive.

If MDMA-assisted therapy gains FDA approval and insurance coverage, it could become accessible to more veterans than ever before. Such a milestone would bring a powerful PTSD treatment into mainstream healthcare and show that psychedelic therapies can meet strict medical standards. Its acceptance could also open the door for psilocybin and other psychedelics to follow, giving veterans more options for healing from trauma.

MDMA-assisted therapy for veteran PTSD

A staggering 71 percent of participants no longer qualified for a PTSD diagnosis after three eight-hour MDMA-assisted therapy sessions. Up to 87 percent experienced clinically significant improvement in their symptoms. Research has shown that MDMA-assisted therapy significantly reduces such PTSD symptoms as nightmares, flashbacks, hypervigilance, and avoidance behaviors in military veterans. These improvements were sustained over time (Mitchell et al., 2021).

————5-MeO-DMT, the "God molecule"————

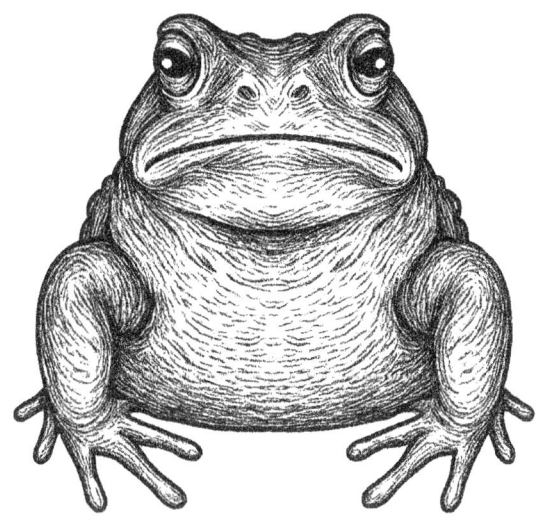

5-MeO-DMT is perhaps the most powerful psychedelic available. Many veterans credit its potency for helping dislodge them from being "stuck" in destructive mental spaces.

One veteran aptly described 5-MeO-DMT as a "nuclear weapon going off." It is four to six times more potent than other forms of DMT and perhaps the most powerful psychedelic available. Many veterans credit its potency for helping dislodge them from being "stuck" in destructive mental spaces.

5-MeO-DMT was traditionally sourced from the venom of the Sonoran Desert Toad (*Bufo alvarius*/*Incilius alvarius*) of the southwestern United States and northwestern Mexico. However, a synthetic version of 5-MeO called "Jaguar" is now commonly favored to spare this imperiled species. Jaguar's dosages are also easier to control than the toad venom. Additionally, 5-MeO can be harvested from the *Anadenanthera peregrina* and *Virola theiodora* plants in Central and South America.

Users typically lose complete awareness of their bodies and their surroundings while in the experience. Many say it is like dying and passing over to the other side without physically dying. This experience of "dying," merging into a universal oneness, and then returning to the body appears to provide profound relief for depression, anxiety, and other states of neurological imprisonment for many participants.

However, because it's so powerful, the experience itself can also induce terror and has the potential to be traumatizing. 5-MeO-DMT should only be done under qualified guidance and with ample preparatory and post-journey support. Additionally, the loss of awareness of oneself and one's surroundings makes supervision necessary to ensure the participant's safety.

The 5-MeO-DMT experience

Because the experience is short and intense, 5-MeO is not typically administered in a group context. The compound is inhaled as a vapor or smoke and takes effect within thirty seconds. The peak occurs between minutes one and fifteen, and the experience lasts about half an hour. It takes another thirty minutes or so to fully reintegrate into the body.

Standard doses of synthetic 5-MeO range from about 8-15 mg, which is comparable to 30–60 mg of toad venom. Some facilitators increase the dose over several rounds, starting with a lower dose and gradually increasing to the full dose.

As mentioned, it's common for people to lose complete awareness of their body, consciousness, and environment during the 5-MeO journey. Participants may fight or resist the experience. Although unaware of this, they sometimes scream, thrash, or yell during this phase. Therefore, it's crucial to have helpers in the room to keep them safe.

When they finally surrender, most users experience profound peace, love, and acceptance, as if they have merged with the universe or a higher power. Users often report that this passage through intense fear and loving surrender is profoundly therapeutic.

People tend to feel completely back to normal after about an hour. However, milder "reactivations," when the 5-MeO effects reoccur to varying degrees, may happen during sleep for about a week after the experience or randomly during the day.

The integration period following a 5-MeO experience can last weeks or months as new revelations continually emerge that need to be processed.

In the veteran community, 5-MeO is often served a day or two after an ibogaine experience. This can help lift someone who may be left feeling beaten down by their ibogaine experience.

5-MeO is often described as a rocket ship that goes into serenity, peace, and unity with God. However, some people have very challenging and terrifying 5-MeO experiences.

The ibogaine–5-MeO combination retreats have become popular in the special operations communities. They can be powerful breakthrough experiences. 5-MeO may be helpful for someone who continually hits walls of feeling stuck and being unable to break through on ayahuasca or psilocybin. 5-MeO can help jettison a person past that resistance so their brain can experience release. At the same time, the experience may be too intense for some people.

With 5-MeO now more easily accessible through vape pens, we worry that such a powerful psychedelic will be used in inappropriate or unsafe settings, with the potential of causing more harm than good.

5-MeO-DMT for veteran PTSD
In one survey, 80 percent of more than 350 respondents reported improvements in anxiety and depression. The degree of improvement was directly related to the intensity of the experience (Wolfgang et al., 2025).

Another study found a decrease in depression and anxiety and an increase in life satisfaction and well-being persisted in a four-week follow-up of 42 participants (Stauffer et al., 2025).

Veteran Voices
Mark Keller
Navy veteran Mark Keller had been a combat fighter pilot before his return to civilian life disintegrated into PTSD, moral injury, and a prescription benzodiazepine addiction. He credits psychedelics, including 5-MeO-DMT, with helping him turn his life around.

"I take this powerful stuff, and it was like a nuclear weapon going off," Keller said.

"I started screaming my head off. It was the most primal scream, but I didn't feel fear. All this heavy, dark stuff that I couldn't bear to face because it was too painful just came out.

"I sit up, still very much under the influence of this medicine, thinking, God, I screwed up another thing. I think I'm quietly apologizing to these guys. 'I'm sorry. I ruined this. I'm not gonna blow it by telling people that sometimes it doesn't work.'

"I didn't realize I was screaming this. And they're like, 'No, man, you're doing great.'

"I think they're patronizing me and hoping I don't jump out of a window or sue them. They lay me back down and put on my eye shades. I was frustrated that I was struggling.

"Then I started to think these guys had set me up, and everyone in the room was in on it. But it was a good form of paranoia. The whole universe was in on it. It was like another nuclear weapon went off.

"I jumped up as I realized that these guys were all in on this plot to get me to understand my purpose. I felt overwhelmed by the power of God's love. I'm not religious, but I was acutely aware that God flows through us and is in all things.

"My chest cracked open, but not in a painful way. It revealed a pure, bright white light inside me, which was God's love shining through me.

"I was running around the room hugging these guys, and I don't mean like, 'Good game, bro.' I mean, like, I love you so deeply I can't find words to describe it. I'm screaming at the top of my lungs, spit flying, crying, 'I love you so much, you can't even understand it. I love you. I love you.'

"I proclaimed at the top of my lungs that my life's purpose is to let people know that God loves us."

Reflecting more than a year later on his experiences, Keller says that no matter how profound your experience is, it's only just the beginning. "Psychedelics kick the door open for healing," he said. "But you gotta walk through the door, and there's a long path for you when you get out.

"Ninety-five percent of it is what you do afterward. But you enjoy this glow for a few months during this period of increased neuroplasticity after a psychedelic journey."

Alex Horton

Alex Horton deployed to Afghanistan with Special Operations as part of the all-women Cultural Support Team. She recalls her 5-MeO-DMT as explosive. "They were giving us smaller doses to ease into it. I remember coming back from the second dose and thinking, I don't wanna go back. Don't make me do that again. And, of course, we immediately went into the next round," she said. "Unbeknownst to me, I locked my jaw open and started screaming at the top of my lungs for twenty minutes. I was trying to fight all these Navy SEALs in the room.

"Everything was just shedding and falling off of me—my family, past stuff with my parents, combat trauma, being queer in America. When I came to, I was ten feet from where I had started, the SEALs were holding me down, and the facilitator, a woman, had her hands on my heart.

"She tried to hold me, and interestingly enough, I needed one of the guys to hug me. He held me, and we just sat there and cried for like ten minutes.

"I needed to shed all those identities and have a man there who'd experienced the same things I had. It felt like he was apologizing to me and forgiving me at the same time. I didn't know I needed that."

Alex credits 5-MeO and her other psychedelic work with opening her up to new ways of being.

"The biggest healing piece for me that I had never felt, and why these medicines are so powerful, is that level of self-love they bring," she said. "That's what I needed, to receive this understanding, like, 'You're good enough.'"

Mescaline and peyote,
─────   ─────
endangered and indigenous

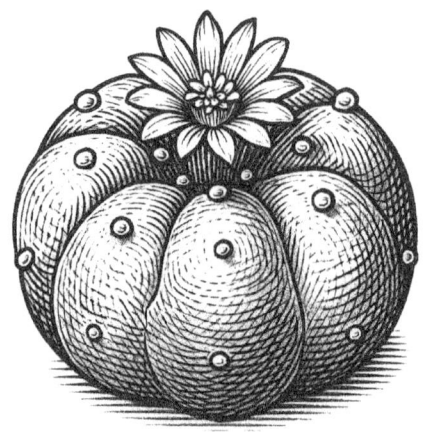

Given its scarcity and spiritual significance among indigenous people of the southwestern U.S. and Mexico, peyote is not widely used in veteran healing communities.

Peyote (*Lophophora williamsii*) is a cactus and was one of the first psychedelics to become popularized in the hippie heyday of psychedelics, thanks partly to Carlos Castaneda's 1968 book *The Teachings of Don Juan: A Yaqui Way of Knowledge*. However, with each peyote button taking ten or more years to mature, that popularity decimated peyote's availability.

In his book *How to Change Your Mind,* author Michael Pollan advocates that non-native people avoid peyote, given its scarcity and spiritual significance among indigenous people of the southwestern U.S. and Mexico.

Traditionally, peyote was used ceremonially among tribes such as the Huichol, Navajo, Comanche, and others to facilitate spiritual experiences, visions, and insights. Today, in the Native American Church, peyote is used to treat drug and alcohol addiction.

Mescaline is the psychoactive compound in peyote and other cacti such as San Pedro and Peruvian Torch. Although isolated mescaline is not commonly found, its effects may differ from those of mescaline-containing cacti.

The peyote/mescaline experience

Mescaline effects are felt within forty-five to ninety minutes of consumption, peaking at two to four hours and lasting for up to eight.

San Pedro, or *huachuma*, grows more quickly than peyote and is easier to access. Journeys tend to be mild compared to other psychedelics.

San Pedro can help one reach deep meditative states with enhanced introspection and emotional exploration. It can also help deepen one's connection to nature. Some San Pedro experts are innovating techniques to make highly potent brews from San Pedro.

Peyote for veteran PTSD

Given its scarcity, peyote is not commonly used among the veteran community. The exception would be for veterans of Native American descent.

PREPARATION, INTEGRATION, AND CHOOSING THE RIGHT SUPPORT

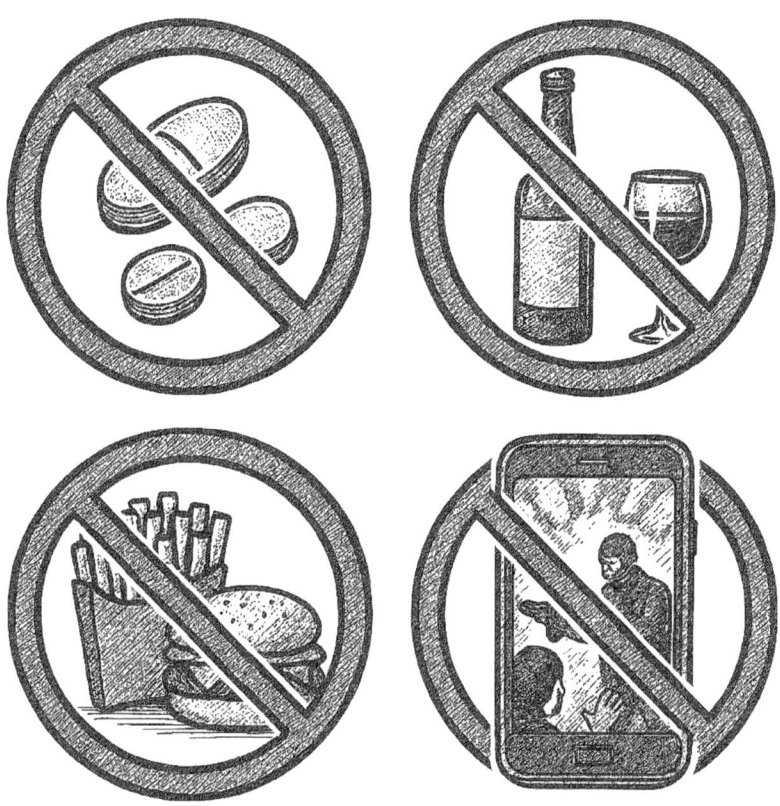

Good preparation is a vital aspect of psychedelic therapy and involves cleansing the mind and body before a journey.

Preparation and integration are vital to psychedelic healing. Both ensure safety and optimize transformative potential. The preparation period enables you to mentally, emotionally, and physically prepare for the journey. The integration period focuses on incorporating the lessons and insights gained from the experience into your life.

————Preparing for a journey————

Preparation through HHP involves individual coaching sessions, group calls, a strict diet, eliminating alcohol, coffee, and other mind-altering substances, and—closer to the journey—abstaining from social media, movies, TV, and sex.

From a logistical standpoint, it also gives HHP time to ensure a person is committed to the process and not just looking for a quick fix. It helps us discern whether any mental health, substance abuse, or medical concerns may make a psychedelic experience inappropriate.

The preparation period begins weeks before any medicine is ingested. The austerity of preparation provides a container for fear, anxiety, contemplation, and any other emotions that may arise. The discipline and focus of preparation foster a sense of reverence amid our busy, distracted lives, which can support the psychedelic experience.

This ceremonial preparation can be likened to entering military life, which involves pre-training, training, and readiness for deployment. The rigor and formality give soldiers a framework for better surviving life-or-death situations. While the psychedelic journey isn't life-threatening, it often involves dismantling long-held internal structures, commonly known as an "ego death." Preparation gives veterans a chance to train for the psychedelic ego death.

————The integration period————

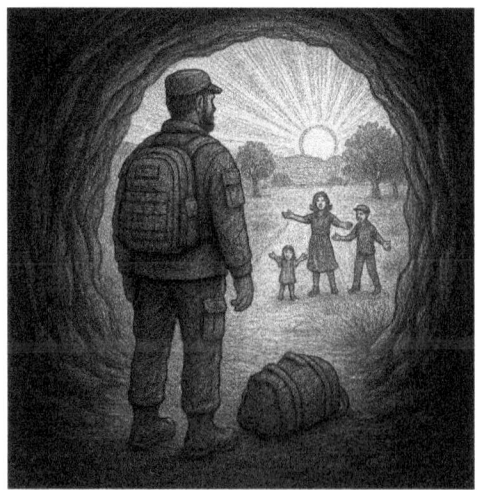

Psychedelic integration involves reflecting on and weaving insights from a psychedelic experience into daily life for healing, growth, and lasting change.

It's essential to follow up a psychedelic journey with strong integration support. While the psychedelic journey is a mystical experience, the integration period is where the magic happens.

Integration looks different for everyone. Many people experience profound breakthroughs that can radically alter their daily lives and lead to new ways of thinking and acting. Suppressed aspects of themselves begin to emerge, which may disrupt their relationships, home lives, or work lives.

Some people have dark or depressing journeys that give them plenty to contemplate, but perhaps leave them feeling cheated or wondering what they did wrong.

Some are teary and emotional after their journey, others jubilant and evangelistic. Some have had profound mystical revelations, but then their rational mind begins to resume its grip, and they start to doubt the experience and its meaning.

Some struggle with massive shifts and need more coaching or therapy than anticipated. Others can take the resources offered to them and implement them to start making changes and creating new connections within the veteran psychedelic community.

HHP's goal is to help people access the post-psychedelic neurological window to start creating new neural pathways and more positive thoughts, habits, and actions. These changes typically do not occur overnight (sometimes they do), but the integration period is the optimal time to begin building those habits. It could be journaling, meditating, regular exercise, cooking, or other positive practices. We aim to help people find something they enjoy practicing and provide group Zoom calls for ongoing mutual support and accountability.

————The importance of community————

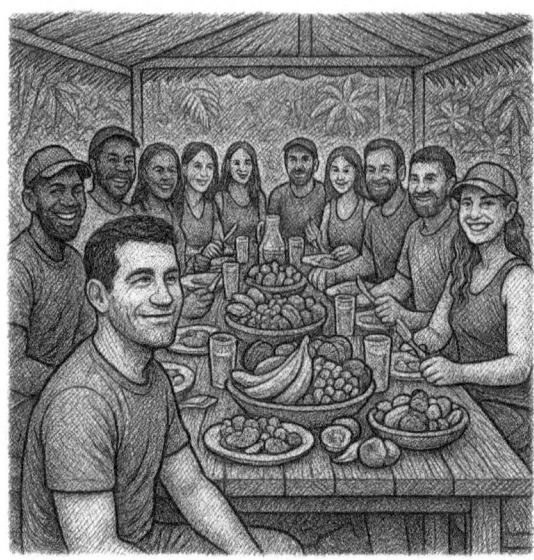

Community is a vital aspect of psychedelic work, especially among veterans who experienced the types of bonds in service that most civilians never do.

Community is a vital aspect of psychedelic work, especially among veterans who experienced the types of bonds in service that most civilians never do. The psychedelic community can help rekindle similar bonds, provide mutual accountability, and allow others to witness our progress or when we might be backsliding and need support.

Religion aside, we can look to churches as an example. They are a way for the local community to check in with one another regularly, maintain communal order and accountability, and provide an opportunity for people to help each other during times of need. The military environment served similar roles for veterans, and they lose this communal infrastructure in civilian life.

Veterans who work with psychedelics find it helpful to be among others who understand both worlds. Veterans often feel the need to censor themselves around civilians, and people who have not worked with psychedelics simply don't have a clue about the experience. When the people around you know where you're coming from, you don't have to guard yourself, explain yourself, or endure well-meaning but unhelpful advice. Even just sitting quietly and listening among your peers can be a powerful aspect of the psychedelic healing process. The most introverted people still need community.

At the same time, some communities can be harmful or destructive. Be wary of cult-like environments with an all-knowing figurehead, cliques, exclusionary behavior, drama, or toxic discussion and behavior. Instead, look for a welcoming, inclusive community focused on positivity and personal evolution.

———Choosing your psychedelic setting and support———

The ideal psychedelic healing environment is a guided group setting with other veterans, led by experienced facilitators. The community, the shared history, and the attention to physical and mental safety are powerful parts of the healing experience. However, we understand this is not available to everyone.

At the time of this writing, it is possible to access legal psilocybin facilitation in Oregon and Colorado. Psychedelic churches throughout the country operate under religious freedom laws. Some cities have decriminalized psychedelics, easing access. You can travel to retreat centers in Central and South America to legally participate in psychedelic ceremonies.

Of course, many people work in illegal underground circles due to the U.S.'s draconian laws around psychedelics. Many of these circles are led by experienced facilitators who adhere to the Indigenous lineages under which they trained. Such circles have benefited countless people, including veterans, for decades.

However, because they operate underground, cases of fraud or abuse can occur without oversight or recourse.

Regardless of your avenue of access, it's essential to be discerning and well-informed when choosing a facilitator, retreat center, and preparation and integration coach.

———Working with a coach———

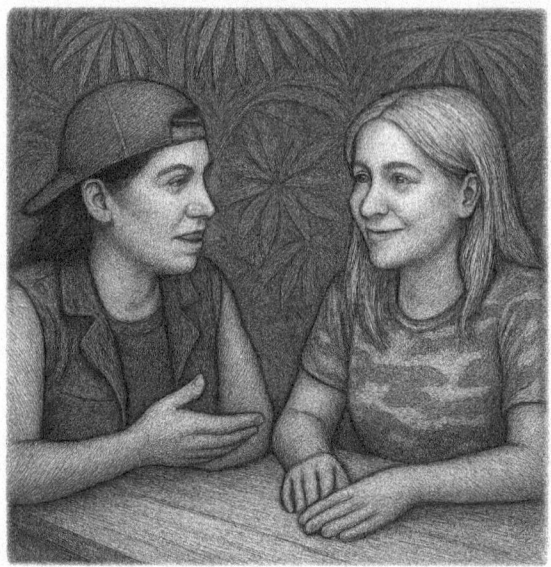

A coach can guide you in translating your journey into tangible changes that foster your growth and evolution.

A good coach will help you distinguish intentions from expectations, navigate challenging feelings and experiences that arise during the preparation period, and assist you in processing the experience.

A coach can also guide you in translating your journey into tangible changes that foster your growth and evolution. This includes helping you stay accountable. Group integration support is also great for accountability.

Screening for good coaches and facilitators:

- Look for individuals with an established background and experience.
- Look for those who align with your values and beliefs.
- Be aware of basic safety and ethical considerations.
- Trust your instincts when meeting a potential facilitator or coach.

Screening for good coaches and facilitators

Choosing experienced coaches and facilitators who "feel" right is important. Word-of-mouth referrals from someone you trust are ideal, but if you don't have any connections, here are some factors to consider:

1. Look for individuals with an established background and experience. Credentials in therapy or counseling are a bonus, though not necessarily indicative of experience. Some uncredentialed experts have been working in psychedelic healing for decades. Your coach or guide should have ample experience working with psychedelics themselves and with others.

2. Look for those who align with your values and beliefs. It's ideal, though not mandatory, to work with a veteran who understands your background.

3. Be aware of basic safety and ethical considerations. You should feel that your autonomy, privacy, and boundaries are respected and not pushed. Ask about their experience working with the emergence of repressed memories or traumas, and supporting people who have had particularly challenging journeys.

4. Trust your instincts when meeting a potential facilitator or coach; your intuition matters profoundly. The success of your relationship depends on trust, respect, and connection. There are many flavors of humans, so take the time to find the right fit for you.

Common pitfalls to be aware of in facilitators and coaches

Good psychedelic facilitation and coaching require putting one's ego in the backseat and navigating the delicate balance between letting someone find their way through a difficult journey and knowing when to offer support.

We see common pitfalls in inexperienced facilitators and coaches:

Over explaining

One pitfall is to "information dump," overloading the participant with tips and how-tos, and then jumping to interpret their experiences. The facilitator or coach should speak the least.

Being overprotective

Inexperienced facilitators often want to shield participants from difficult experiences. A facilitator's job is to help prepare participants, provide a safe container, and be available for help, but not to "rescue" a participant from a tough spot.

Blaming the participant for not "letting go"

One of the most harmful myths we see perpetuated in psychedelic spaces is the idea that someone had a challenging journey because they are "blocked" or unable to "let go."While these are genuine challenges that can arise, it's important not to put the onus on the individual or make them feel at fault, as if they did psychedelics "wrong." That's like telling someone with clinical depression to cheer up, or encouraging someone with an anxiety disorder to relax.

The psyche of someone new to psychedelics, who came of age in military culture or combat, may equate letting go with a death sentence.

Navigating blocks may be a matter of working with an experienced guide, developing familiarity with psychedelics, using a different psychedelic, or perhaps finding another avenue of help. We want to remind people regularly that while we advocate for veteran access to psychedelic therapy, this path is not appropriate for everyone.

Qualities to consider in a retreat center

Many people travel to psychedelic retreat centers in Central and South America. Look for personal referrals from a trusted source when possible.

Consider these factors in a retreat center:

- What safety precautions are in place?
- What is the ratio of facilitators and helpers to participants?
- How were the retreat experience and ceremonies developed? Is there an indigenous lineage? Is the relationship with the indigenous healers equitable or exploitative?
- How is the medicine prepared?

The retreat center should be transparent and forthcoming with its information. Trust your impressions and your sense of the people involved. If you sense bravado and ego that rubs you the wrong way, pay attention to that.

It's essential to look for baseline safety, reverence, and professionalism in all areas of psychedelic treatment. At the same time, avoid the temptation to search for perfection or be overly detailed with your inquiries. It's ok to ask for the ingredients in a restaurant dish, but you don't need to know the name of the farm the chicken came from.

CHAPTER 14

THE RISKS OF PSYCHEDELIC THERAPY

Psychiatric drugs often work by suppressing symptoms; people complain they feel "numb." Psychedelics do the opposite. They can suddenly bring to the surface aspects of their psyches that have been in the shadows for years or decades. Just as each person's genetic makeup can dictate how their body will uniquely respond to a medication, so a psychological fingerprint can make it challenging to predict how they will respond to psychedelics.

Except for the accepted psychological diagnostic framework, we don't have assessment tools to determine a person's risk or resilience in psychedelic treatment.

This is why we heavily emphasize support structures for preparation and integration. Attention to both makes a profound difference in how safely and effectively one navigates the psychedelic therapy journey.

In this chapter, we will explore the potential risks and challenges of psychedelic use. While most participants do not experience adverse effects, it is essential to approach your journey with full awareness and understanding.

Hallucinogen Persisting Perception Disorder (HPPD)
Hallucinogen Persisting Perception Disorder (HPPD) is a rare but potentially long-lasting condition characterized by visual disturbances following psychedelic use. Although it occurs most frequently with LSD, it can also arise from other psychedelics and is thought to affect the brain's visual processing. The severity and duration of HPPD can vary, with some cases persisting indefinitely without full resolution.

Symptoms may include seeing visual snow, images after they're no longer in view, halos around objects, trails behind moving objects, flashes, and size distortion of objects.

——A challenging integration period——

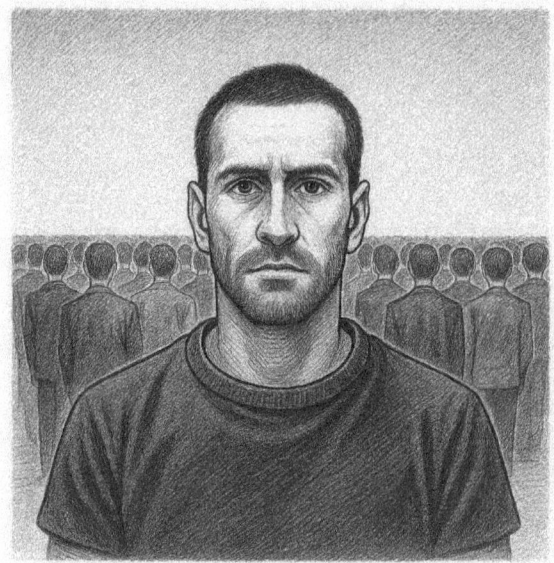

While many people experience an afterglow following a psychedelic journey, sometimes it can be a difficult period.

When repressed memories surface during a psychedelic journey, they need care and attention. Such memories can reveal patterns the person may never have fully understood, but they can also shake up how they see themselves. It often takes time to work through the emotions these memories stir up and to weave those revelations into an evolving identity.

During the journey, people sometimes realize they have unwittingly become accustomed to toxic or destructive jobs, relationships, or situations. With this newfound clarity, they recognize that they must make significant life changes to break free from these unhealthy patterns.

For others, the psychedelic journey was so expansive and revolutionary that being plunked back into daily life feels jarring and disorienting.

We encourage veterans to lean heavily on group calls and other forms of integration support during these periods. We also advise people to trust that they will begin to feel more grounded after a few weeks.

If people pursue subsequent journeys, they know what to expect and often enjoy the profound insights and revelations that occur during the psychedelic "afterglow."

While the "real world" can feel discombobulating during the post-journey period, this is also when feelings of unconditional love, inner peace, and deep trust in the universe or a higher power are often at their strongest. This heightened spiritual connection can offer profound comfort and guidance during the integration process.

However, if you are feeling untethered and more anxious after your journey, we suggest working with a mental health care professional.

Psychedelic hucksters, cult leaders, and opportunists

A surge in the popularity of psychedelic healing has attracted predatory and opportunistic people, making it important to be alert to red flags.

For instance, some businesses or facilitators promote psychedelics with exaggerated claims or guaranteed results. While psychedelics can lead to profound healing, reputable centers and facilitators avoid misleading people with overblown promises. Instead, they provide a balanced view, emphasizing that outcomes vary and that the healing process requires integration, support, and holding realistic expectations.

Another trap to be wary of is cult-like leaders or communities founded around the personalities of their leaders. When uniformity of language, behavior, or ideology is required for belonging, and non-conformity is shamed or shunned, it may not create a positive or supportive environment.

Unfortunately, some psychedelic facilitators are downright harmful, exploiting the vulnerability of the psychedelic experience to manipulate or abuse participants, whether financially, emotionally, or sexually. Always do your research and, if possible, seek referrals from trusted individuals to ensure a safe and supportive environment.

Psychedelics and narcissistic personality tendencies

A common refrain in the psychedelic space is, "If every government leader and corporate executive did psychedelics, the world would be a better place." Most people do become more open-minded and open-hearted when working with psychedelics. However, we have seen exceptions to this.

Although no formal research has been conducted on the effects of psychedelics on narcissistic personality disorder (NPD) or self-aggrandizing personalities, many anecdotal reports suggest that psychedelics can exacerbate these traits. While most people are humbled when encountering ego dissolution and universal consciousness, those with narcissistic tendencies may interpret these experiences as affirming their superiority or divine status. NPD traits, along with a fixation on power, are often seen in political leaders and corporate executives, and psychedelics may heighten these tendencies in some. Although this is based on casual observation and not scientific evidence, it remains an important consideration.

Psychedelics help many people connect more deeply with their authentic selves, but saying they will make the world a better place may be overly optimistic.

———Taking "orders" from the medicine———

People sometimes receive profound direction during their journeys, which can be inspiring and productive. For example, they may adopt healthier habits, make amends with someone, or start working towards something they've always dreamed of.

However, when the medicine "tells you" to quit your job, leave your spouse, sell all your belongings, move into a van, burn all your journals, or make other drastic changes, we ask people to give those decisions at least a thirty-day probation period. Sometimes, the messages that come through ecstatic moments are simply bouts of fantasy or impulsivity. You'll likely be grateful that you gave yourself a cooling-off period and didn't devastate your security or stability. If you need to change aspects of your life, proceed from a more grounded and patient state of mind.

————Getting stuck in victim mode————

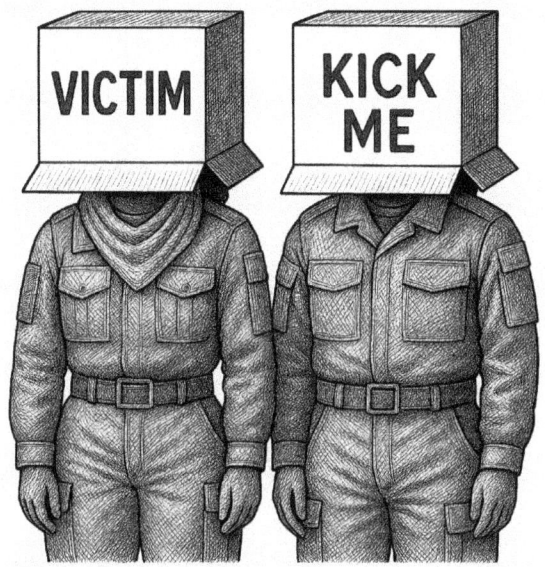

It's common for mental health disorders to foster a sense of victimhood. One must be willing to move past this when working with psychedelics or MDMA.

Many individuals who have struggled for years with PTSD, depression, or suicidal ideation often find themselves stuck in a victim mentality. This isn't meant to be disparaging or shaming; when your neurology is locked down, it can feel like you're trapped in inescapable patterns of thought.

However, we sometimes encounter people who are unwilling or unable to shift from a victim mentality to a more personal sense of agency. People trapped in this pattern see themselves singled out for life's misfortunes. If this appears as a strong trait during the intake period, it may disqualify a person for psychedelic therapy.

That's because they are more likely to interpret any challenges that arise as personal attacks, make the psychedelic journey the new source of all their problems, or double down on their trauma, rather than seeking a way through it.

These individuals may have a profound breakthrough experience but revert to their old ways once the afterglow wears off, and refuse to use the integration tools or support offered.

Again, we say this not to blame or shame but to point out that these individuals may benefit more from other therapeutic approaches.

———Post-journey depression———

People rarely become more depressed or even suicidal after their journey, but we'd be remiss to ignore that it occasionally happens. If a psychedelic journey unearths long-repressed traumas or memories, it may overwhelm a person to the point of despair.

It's tempting to believe that the post-journey afterglow is your new operating system. While the journey has lasting effects, the afterglow is a two- to three-week honeymoon period. It offers a window of clarity and openness, but it's essentially the "training wheels" before you begin integrating the insights and lessons.

Some become frantic or fearful of going back to their old ways. This is understandable, primarily if you subconsciously built your lifestyle and relationships around supporting your trauma responses. However, the psychedelic experience introduces new insights and inner tools that weren't previously available. Using these is where the work begins to rewire the brain. Practicing self-love, trust, and feeling safe can be challenging when you haven't felt those things in years or possibly ever. The psychedelic experience may immerse you in these positive states, offering your brain a blueprint to follow as you work toward lasting change.

Also, not everyone has a honeymoon period. Some may emerge feeling more depressed, lethargic, or unsure. This, too, is normal and, again, typically stems from unresolved mental gunk coming to the surface.

While psychedelics help many people become more positive and fully-realized versions of themselves, at the end of the day, you are still you. The goal is not to become someone different but to befriend and champion who you already are.

Coming home to a toxic environment
built around perpetuating trauma

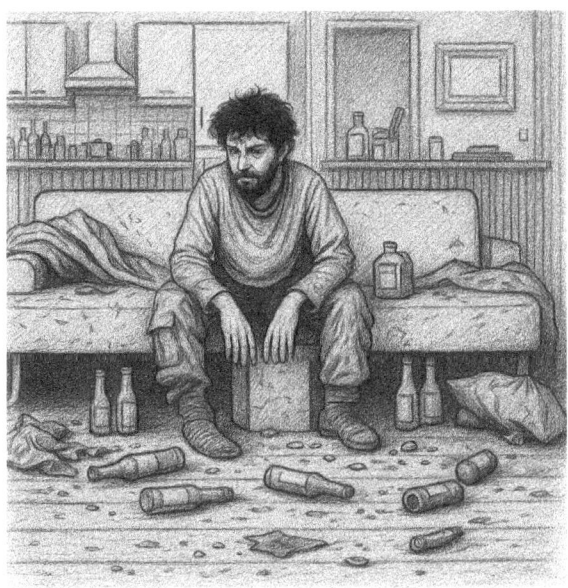

Returning to an environment you unconsciously created to perpetuate your trauma can hinder progress. It's an aspect of recovery you must address.

Trauma often leads us to unconsciously create relationships, social circles, environments, and routines that perpetuate our trauma. A psychedelic journey may be eye-opening and healing, but if you return to an environment you unwittingly created to perpetuate your trauma, you have that much more healing work to do. This can trigger depression or anxiety.

Just as we unconsciously build routines and lifestyles to feed trauma, so can we consciously create them to feed healing.

We acknowledge the significant challenges in dismantling old dynamics, setting boundaries, and walking away from destructive situations so that you can create a more positive life.

We advocate making changes little by little while coming to terms with what you need and getting support to process the feelings that arise.

For many people, the insights gained in the psychedelic journey are the first of many small steps on a lifelong path. We often hear from participants a year later that breaking free of these patterns is one of the hardest things they've done, but also the most healing and rewarding.

Developing psychological
dependence on psychedelics

Psychedelics are not addictive despite their erroneous Schedule 1 classification. In fact, the psychedelic journey can be so psychologically and emotionally intense that most people need ample breaks between journeys and can't imagine "abusing" a psychedelic. But let's face it: the monotony and pressures of daily life are nowhere near as interesting as a psychedelic journey.

The psychedelic-assisted healing transformation requires work and a willingness to embrace challenge. Rather than face that, some people return repeatedly to the psychedelic realm. They become dependent on the sensations of an alternate reality, the fantastical visuals, the extreme experiences, and the ego boost of taking ever larger "heroic" doses. They may defend this practice by arguing that ordinary reality is corrupt or fake.

Thankfully, we have not seen this happen often. Most people find meaning in their lives thanks to their psychedelic healing work.

While we respect that there is more than one psychedelic path, HHP's stance is that psychedelics help us better participate in life and not escape from it.

Walking the psychedelic path
is not all sunshine and roses

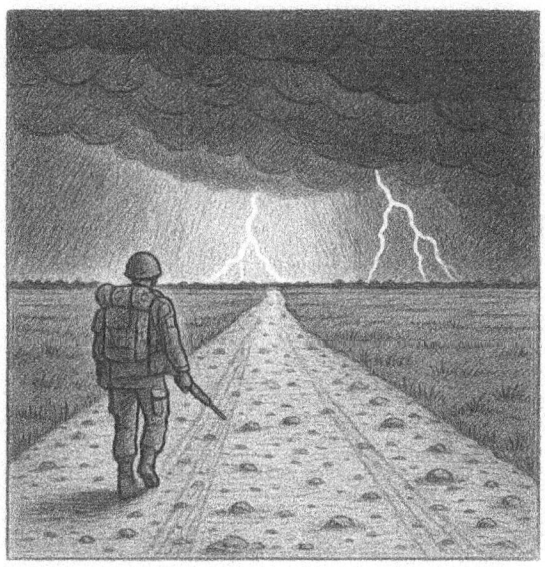

Psychedelic healing does not mean you live happily ever after.
It requires time, patience, and active commitment.

Many people in Western culture grow up without an emphasis on self-re-flection and mindfulness. As a result, we can spend decades repressing dif-ficult yet essential aspects of ourselves. The psychedelic experience has a way of illuminating these hidden parts, which can shake or even shatter the foundations of our psychological framework. When this happens, we must consciously rebuild this framework, which can be rewarding but disruptive, much like tilling the soil for a more abundant harvest.

This is why we strongly emphasize the importance of preparation and inte-gration. Unlike a pharmaceutical approach, which often focuses on symptom suppression, psychedelic healing delves deeper, addressing root causes and requiring time, patience, and active commitment. For this reason, it is not something to be taken lightly.

CHAPTER 15

BAD TRIPS

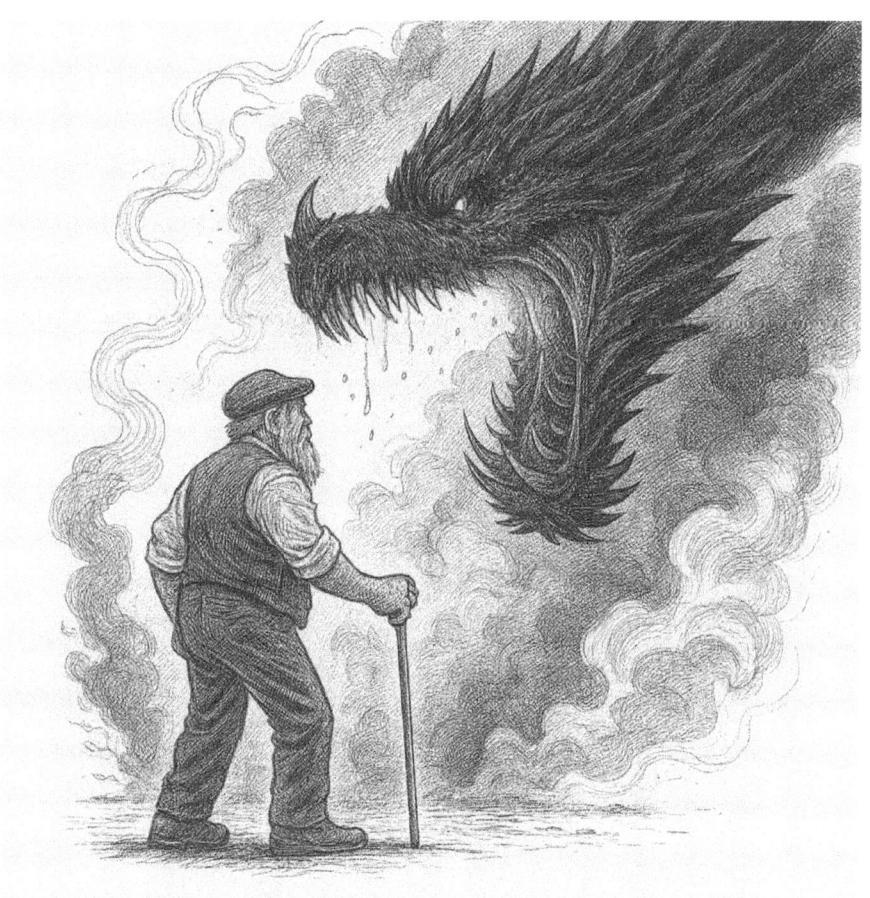

Bad trips happen. They can be instructive, but there are also ways to mitigate their occurrence.

While psychedelic trip reports frequently include visits with God and dissolution into eternal love, sometimes bad trips happen. A bad trip can consist of feeling terror, isolation, or despair, feeling trapped in a mental loop, feeling you are about to die, horrific mental images, or other profoundly distressing emotions, sensations, and experiences.

Psychedelics plunge us into the deep end of the human experience, which includes exaltation, joy, terror, anxiety, monotony, stillness, agitation, bliss, and so on.

These experiences help us better understand and navigate the internal worlds that inevitably arise in "the real world." Although we naturally prefer ecstatic journeys, it's important to recognize that all experiences hold value and opportunity for self-understanding, even the challenging ones (many would argue, *especially* the challenging ones).

That said, you don't have to have a bad trip to heal. Also, not all difficult experiences are "bad." Journeys can include tours through grief and loss, the emergence of repressed memories, or re-experiencing past traumas. Most participants do not consider these "bad trips," but deeply therapeutic experiences that ultimately brought them greater peace.

Bad trips tend to land more in the sphere of anxiety, panic, fear, despair, or horror. However, you can employ various strategies to reduce the potential for a bad trip.

Six ways to reduce the potential for a bad trip:

1. Secure your "set and setting."

2. Practice relaxation techniques ahead of time so you can deploy them automatically.

3. Hydrate, be well rested, and balance blood sugar.

4. Avoid an overly large dose your first time.

5. Clear your schedule.

6. Lean into it.

---

1. Secure your "set and setting."

"Set and setting" is a common term in the psychedelic world. "Set" refers to your mental landscape, and "setting" refers to the location and environment of your journey. It's important to prepare both carefully before your journey.

Common ways to optimize your mindset several weeks before a journey include following a cleansing diet, avoiding mind-altering substances, reducing media and social media consumption, and reflecting on your intentions. Ideally, this period also involves working with a coach or therapist and participating in group calls with other participants.

Your setting deserves careful attention as well. Many bad trips happen at festivals and concerts where there is too much stimulation that overwhelms the mind. Your setting should be secure, comfortable, quiet, and designed to support your well-being. Having a qualified facilitator or trip sitter present is important for safety and to enhance feelings of security. In addition to a lead facilitator, a group setting will also have several helpers on hand so anyone who needs support has it.

Music is an important accompaniment to psychedelic journeys. Music at a retreat is carefully chosen to guide participants throughout the journey. If you provide your own music, screen playlists on Spotify or other streaming sources to ensure no ads pop up, and that you don't find any of the music agitating.

2. Practice relaxation techniques ahead of time so you can deploy them automatically.

Choose relaxation techniques that appeal to you and practice them regularly before your journey. This will make it natural to employ them should you begin to feel overwhelmed. Calming breathing techniques such as box breathing, alternate nostril breathing, and longer exhales are effective and versatile. Other ideas include relaxing your face, changing your position, and moving your body to release trapped energy.

3. Hydrate, be well rested, and balance blood sugar.

Before your journey, support your brain with good hydration and nutrition that stabilizes your blood sugar and mood. Do your best to arrive for your journey well-rested.

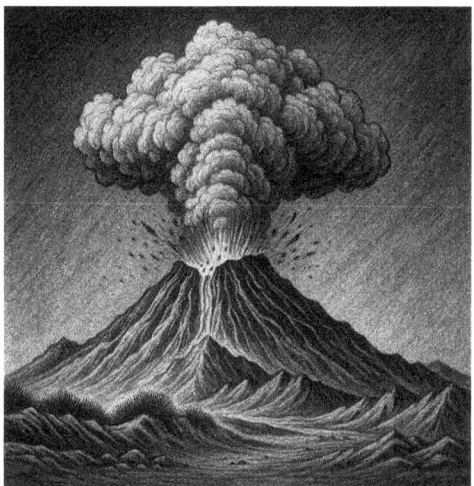

The psychedelic journey is no place for a big ego. The heroic dose is not advised for beginners with significant trauma.

4. Avoid an overly large dose for your first trip.

In psychedelic lingo, a "heroic dose" simply means a large dose. While breaking into a mystical experience can be where the magic happens, leave your ego at the door when it comes to your dose. Too much too soon can be unnecessarily overwhelming. Most retreats will determine your dose for you and avoid giving newcomers overly large doses. If you're given an option, start conservatively, especially if you have the option to take a second dose an hour or two into the journey. It is always easier to take more, but you can't untake a psychedelic once it's ingested or inhaled.

5. Clear your schedule.

Clear your calendar so you do not have any obligations immediately after your journey. If you must go to work, travel, or attend an event a day or two after your journey, this may introduce anxiety. Thinking about real-world obligations during your journey may feel overwhelming or intrusive. Instead, give yourself the freedom to fully immerse yourself in the experience without the pressure of impending responsibilities.

Additionally, psychedelics can leave you feeling emotionally and physically sensitive after the experience. Give yourself a few days post-journey to buffer yourself from the "real world" and process your experience.

6. Lean into it.

Sometimes, the best way out of a bad trip is through it. It's natural to tense up, resist, and fight when fear, anxiety, panic, or other challenging experiences arise. Although it's easier said than done, sometimes the best way out of a bad trip is to submit to it. Lean into the awfulness with a willingness to meld with it. This can sometimes neutralize a bad trip and is what people mean by "letting go." Conversely, some people more experienced with psychedelics may feel a bad trip coming on and simply divert it with a thought like, "Not today," or "Not interested."

From bliss to terror, the mind can create fantastically powerful states at either end of the spectrum. The goal isn't to overpower or tame the mind as one must do in survival situations, but rather to get to know, befriend, and support it.

CHAPTER 16

VETERANS ARE LEADING THE PSYCHEDELIC HEALING MISSION

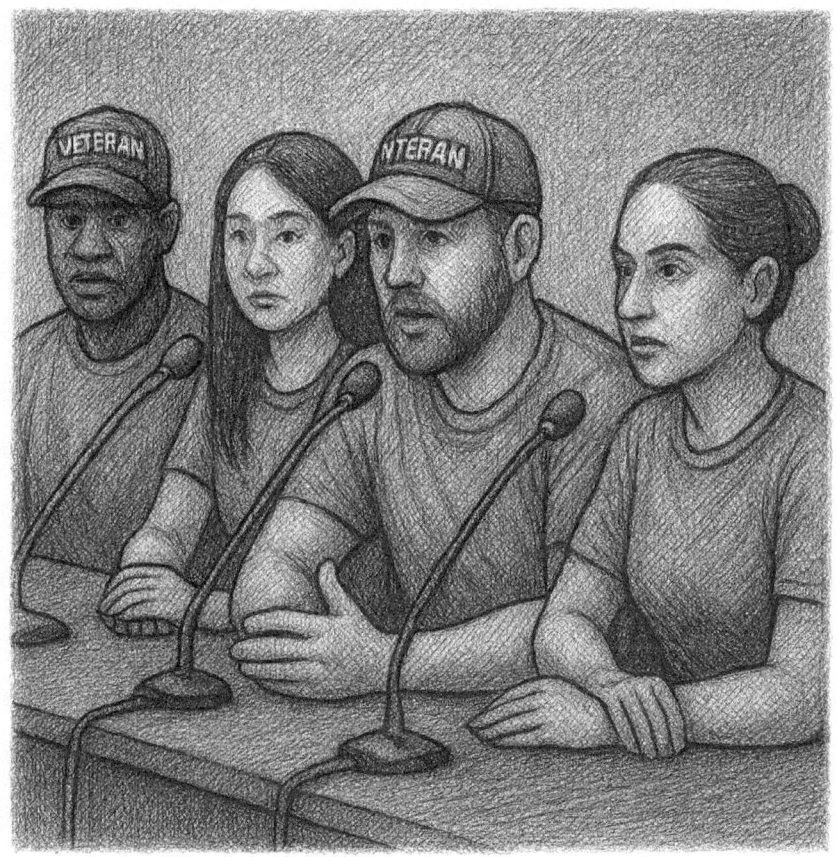

Veterans are at the forefront of one of the most strategic advocacy campaigns in modern drug policy history.

Psychedelic therapy for veterans began as an underground response to their suicide and mental health crisis. Private ayahuasca circles, underground veteran facilitators, and a growing number of veteran-focused retreat centers in less restrictive countries like Mexico built the movement through word of mouth.

Meanwhile, because Schedule I status effectively blocks federal research grants in the U.S., psychedelic and MDMA studies have relied heavily on private donations, with increasing attention directed toward veterans. This strategy serves several purposes: it addresses a population with disproportionately high rates of PTSD, suicide, and other mental health challenges; it frames these therapies as responses to an urgent crisis; it builds bipartisan political support; and amplifies awareness within the veteran community. While formal research has involved only a limited number of veterans, countless others have sought out these therapies independently.

The result? One of the most strategic advocacy campaigns in modern drug policy history is underway. Veterans have historically had to fight through grassroots movements to heal the wounds of war. Psychedelic advocacy is simply the latest chapter in that ongoing battle, and it happens to be an effective lever for policy reform. Veterans are uniquely positioned to bridge political divides and command the attention of lawmakers to a degree that other advocacy groups cannot.

As Marine Corps veteran Juliana Mercer, who leads HHP's federal advocacy efforts, explains, "No one is going to listen to me as a woman. They're not going to listen to me as a person of color. But they're going to listen to me as a veteran."

Mercer leads advocacy efforts for Healing Breakthrough, HHP's policy partner that works directly with the VA and Congress to secure legal medical access to psychedelic and MDMA therapy for veterans. Jason Moore-Brown, an Army veteran who played a prominent role in expanding cannabis rights, focuses on state-level policy reform. Together, they advocate for veterans at both the national and state levels to expand access.

What stands in the way of psychedelic healing for veterans?

Despite ample scientific evidence and increasing political support, multiple barriers, such as stigma, lack of awareness, and limited funding, continue to block veterans' access to these potentially life-saving treatments.

The stigma around psychedelics

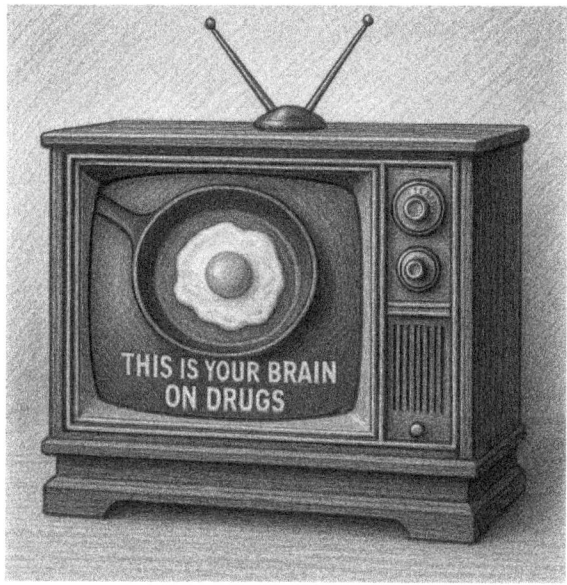

*Stigma rooted in the Vietnam War era continues to shape misguided
drug laws, silencing one of the most promising tools for healing.*

The campaign to stigmatize psychedelics during the Vietnam War persists today, despite decades of evidence for their therapeutic use.

While organized resistance has come from a few special interest groups, response from lawmakers is what Mercer describes as "overwhelmingly and surprisingly positive." Many have been tracking the veteran suicide crisis since the post-9/11 wars and are also frustrated with the poor recovery rate of conventional treatments. "When I show up in their offices with a sci-ence-based solution for PTSD, they have a much easier time being open to a new approach," says Mercer.

The most significant barrier comes from federal regulations that categorized psychedelics as Schedule I drugs: LSD and psilocybin in 1970 and MDMA in 1985. Schedule I classification means substances have "no currently accepted medical use" and "high potential for abuse." This federal classifica-tion can override loosening state laws at any time, creating legal uncertainty in states that have passed decriminalization measures.

Even in progressive states like California, comprehensive psychedelic therapy bills have failed multiple times. As Moore-Brown explains, the state passed decriminalization through both chambers of the legislature only to have Governor Gavin Newsom veto the bill (which had bipartisan support), reportedly due to his presidential ambitions. The following year, a more narrowly focused bill that addressed the governor's concerns didn't make it out of one chamber. "Veterans, regardless of how important our issues are, are still subject to politics, just like every other issue," says Moore-Brown.

The deeply rooted stigma also prevents advocates from talking about LSD altogether, despite its breakthrough therapy designation, because of persistent myths about people running through the streets naked or jumping off rooftops. Meanwhile, alcohol, which kills about 178,000 Americans each year and leads to many acts of violence, domestic abuse, and car crashes, remains not only legal but also deeply ingrained in American culture, exposing the arbitrary and hypocritical nature of our drug scheduling system.

Difficulty raising awareness among veterans
Contrary to popular belief, there's no "veteran hub" through which to dispatch new treatments or requests for research participants. Veterans are often geographically dispersed, returning to rural communities with limited resources.

"The biggest problem, no matter what veteran issue you're working on, is finding the veterans," says Mercer.

Limited Research and Funding
At the time of this writing, the VA has made significant progress in psychedelic research. In 2024, the VA allocated a modest—by research standards—$1.5 million toward an MDMA-assisted therapy study and issued a call for proposals for additional psychedelic research.

The following year, the VA Secretary publicly announced support for psychedelic and MDMA therapy. However, funding remains a primary constraint. Veteran advocacy organizations, which run on donations, have a limited lobbying budget and ability to compete against well-funded opposition.

While these developments offer concrete hope, they've only just gotten the movement across the starting line. Transforming federal policy and expanding access will require sustained political pressure, funding, and continued bipartisan support to overturn decades of punitive regulatory barriers.

The ultimate barrier may be time itself. As Jason Moore-Brown notes, with approximately 6,000 veteran suicides happening annually, each delay in access represents lives lost that could have been saved.

The strategy for moving forward

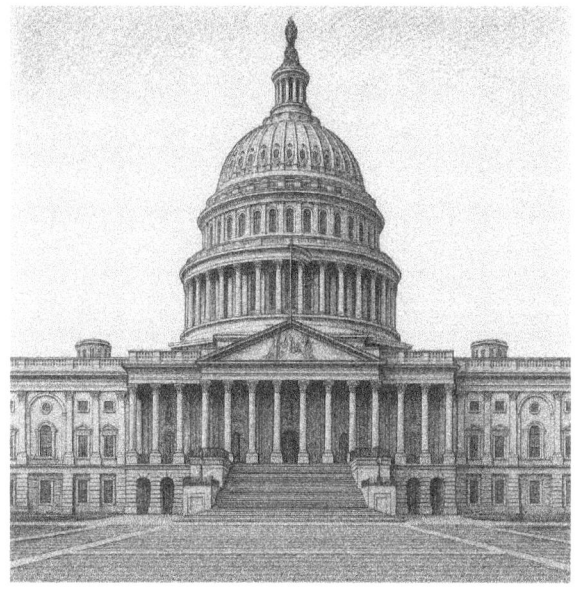

As long as psychedelics remain classified as Schedule I substances, the battle to expand veteran access to this healing therapy is just beginning.

Cultural acceptance of psychedelics skyrocketed after the publication of Michael Pollan's 2018 book *How to Change Your Mind*, which became a Netflix series in 2022. This catalyzed an explosion of psychedelic societies, retreats, advocacy, funding, and more research.

However, as long as psychedelics remain classified as Schedule I substances, the real battle is only beginning. The veteran movement to expand access, which is led by HHP and such veteran organizations as Veterans Exploring Treatment Solutions (VETS), Plant Medicine Coalition, Reason for Hope, Veteran Mental Health Leadership Coalition, requires a multi-pronged strategy at the local and federal levels.

At the federal level, advocates like Mercer focus on supporting VA research and securing congressional appropriations, while state-level organizers, such as Moore-Brown, work to create local access and build political momentum.

Federal efforts help legitimize psychedelic treatments, while state-level victories demonstrate that psychedelic therapy can work in a legal setting. For example, Oregon became the first state to legalize psilocybin service centers in 2020, followed by decriminalization measures in Colorado and several other states. As advocates watch these pioneering programs unfold, they adapt and refine the models for their own regions. Eventually, these approaches become blueprints for how to serve the broader population and integrate psychedelic and MDMA therapies into existing healthcare systems.

Leading with "low-hanging fruit"

The movement has been prioritizing MDMA and psilocybin while avoiding discussion of other psychedelics, even those with breakthrough therapy designations. Leading with what Mercer calls "the low-hanging fruit" has accelerated the acceptance and implementation of policy changes.

This approach helps establish credibility before moving on to lesser-understood substances like LSD and ibogaine, even though ibogaine shows profound potential for treating opiate addiction.

For instance, in 2024, with the help of VETS and Texans for Greater Mental Health, Texas created the largest state-funded psychedelic research program in U.S. history with the Texas Ibogaine Initiative. The program allocates up to $50 million in public funding, matched by equal private investment for FDA-approved clinical trials studying ibogaine's effectiveness in treating opioid use disorder, PTSD, and traumatic brain injury in veterans and first responders.

The opioid crisis affects not only veterans but an alarming number of Americans. It was veteran-led psychedelic advocacy that secured bipartisan support to study a federally illegal compound. Additionally, this public-private partnership funding model gives Texas a commercial stake in any resulting intellectual property, serving as a template for other states to both fund research and generate revenue for veteran services.

Focusing on the data

Thanks to the sustained efforts of MAPS and private fundraising, decades of research, much of it focused on veterans, has quietly built a body of evidence that is increasingly shifting public and legislative opinion. This strategy emphasizes scientific data over emotional appeal. When Mercer meets with state legislators, she leads with hard statistics, forcing skeptics to argue against empirical evidence rather than rely on decades-old propaganda or bias.

A data-driven strategy works because it addresses lawmakers' frustration with failed solutions for the veteran mental health and suicide crisis. "Legislators have been trying to solve this problem for the last two decades, throwing everything at the wall to see if anything sticks," Mercer says. "Nothing has worked because we still have 6,000 veterans dying by suicide each year.' At the same time, veteran voices and stories carry weight. Veterans played a key role in the passage of Oregon's Psilocybin Services Act and in persuading some counties not to opt out of the measure. Veterans like Mercer and Moore-Brown understand they're leveraging their service credentials to open doors that might otherwise remain closed. "If I hadn't been a veteran, I probably wouldn't have gotten any meetings, and I don't think I would have been taken as seriously as I have been," Moore-Brown says.

Building bipartisan support

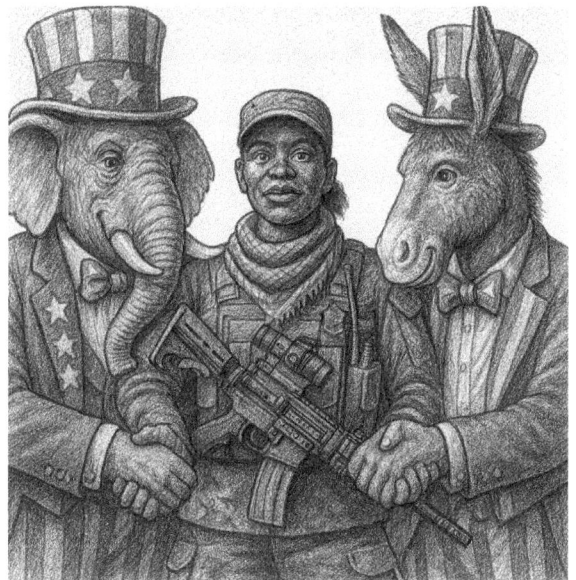

The political diversity within the veteran community, paired with genuine concern for veteran well-being, has made psychedelic therapy a uniquely bipartisan cause.

While Democrats are seen as generally more receptive to psychedelic therapies, Mercer says people might be surprised at how receptive Republicans are as well. The political diversity within the veteran community, paired with genuine concern for veteran well-being, has made psychedelic therapy a uniquely bipartisan cause. Notable veteran politicians who have supported these initiatives include Rep. Jack Bergman (R-MI), Rep. Dan Crenshaw (R-TX), and Rep. Morgan Luttrell (R-TX), while VA Under Secretary for Health Dr. Shereef Elnahal and former Texas Governor Rick Perry have also championed expanded access to psychedelic treatments for veterans.

"We have veterans coming together from all parts of the political spectrum," says Mercer. "This isn't about political affiliation, it's about bringing a solution that can help save lives."

The VA as the primary target

The Department of Veterans Affairs has emerged as an optimal hub for researchers, physicians, and healthcare professionals open to exploring psychedelic and MDMA therapies. It offers a controlled testing environment, a clearly defined patient population with urgent needs, and the potential to serve as a national model.

Ongoing advocacy efforts include supporting VA-led research through public–private funding partnerships, securing congressional appropriations for psychedelic studies, and fostering relationships with VA innovators advancing MDMA, ketamine, and other psychedelic therapies.

The necessity of sustained pressure

Perhaps most importantly, the strategy recognizes that lasting change demands sustained pressure, not just isolated wins. Setbacks are inevitable, and even victories may be partial or symbolic. "Until we get long-term resolutions to the veteran suicide, mental health, and substance abuse issues we're currently facing, veterans will continue to lead the charge," says Moore-Brown.

Why veterans are natural advocates

As discussed throughout this book, veteran culture remains distinct from civilian society long after service ends. It's marked by the ethos of both self-reliance and "leave no man behind" that drove the underground spread of psychedelic therapies. As Moore-Brown explains, veterans were "trained to not sit passively awaiting orders." When they recognized that the government was not going to solve the suicide crisis, they did what they've always done: found solutions through their own networks and took care of each other.

However, Mercer warns that while veteran voices are critical to expanding access to psychedelic and MDMA therapies, their own healing should always come first. When veterans begin on the psychedelic healing path, many find they go through a profound but delicate period of transformation when the brain is repatterning, relationships are shifting, habits are changing, and a rekindled sense of purpose is emerging. This intense period of transformation should be cherished and protected. Going too public too soon may interrupt this fragile process, jeopardizing the healing process.

"You don't owe anything to this movement," says Mercer. "You are healing, and taking care of yourself is the most important thing that you could possibly do. You don't need to advocate." Driven by the same sense of mission that compelled them to enlist, many veterans become psychedelic facilitators and coaches, or advocates who encourage former teammates who are struggling to pursue psychedelic therapy. Most people who attend retreats go because a friend encouraged them. This organic spread of life-saving information reflects a fundamental aspect of military culture that Mercer calls the "Lance Corporal Underground" in the Marines, and Moore-Brown refers to it as the "E-4 Mafia" in the Army. These are informal networks where lower ranks serve as the go-to for practical knowledge.

"The veteran community has always been really good at sharing what's good, what works, and what's bad, what doesn't work, and who to trust and who not to trust," explains Mercer. "When you need an answer, you go to that lower rank, and you ask them what's going on because they know everything and how to get things done."

Psychedelic and MDMA therapy for veterans will always travel through these trusted military networks. No matter what happens in Washington, veterans will continue to find and share what works to save each other's lives.

CHAPTER 17

A VISION FOR THE FUTURE: A NEW MODEL FOR VETERAN COMMUNITIES

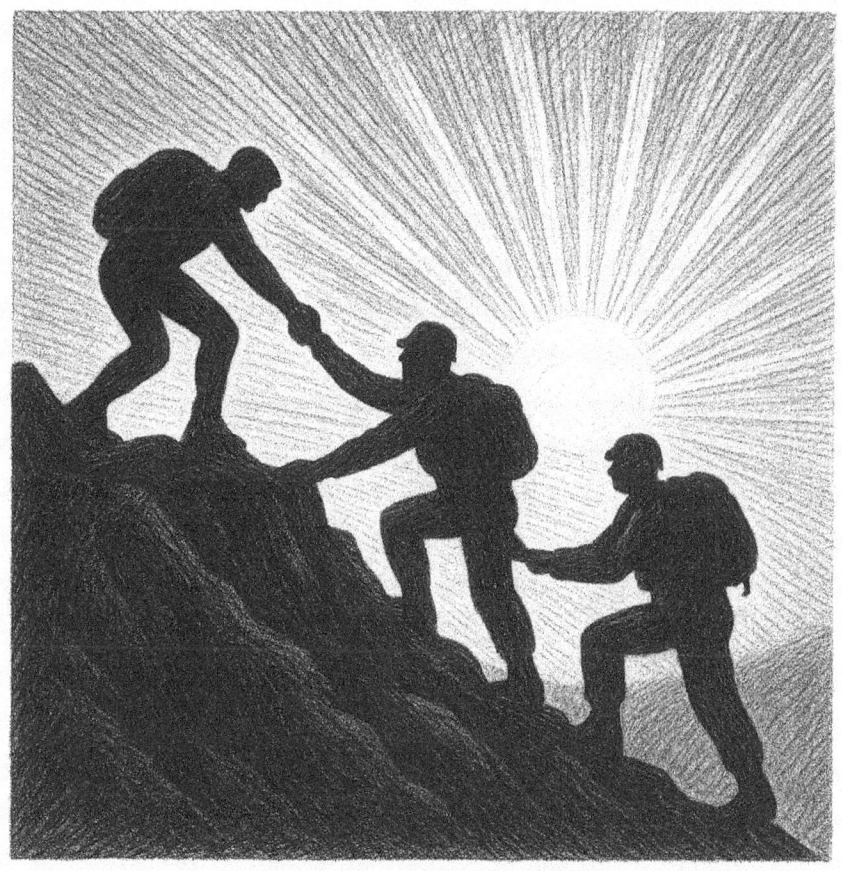

Veterans need spaces where they can be fully themselves, where their military identity is honored rather than pathologized, and where they can build meaningful connections.

Humans are inherently social creatures, and healing often happens best in a community. Long before PTSD was recognized as a medical diagnosis, veterans instinctively gathered in groups to support one another. This pattern mirrors other successful healing communities, like Alcoholics Anonymous, which provides structure and support without central authority.

Traditional veteran gathering spaces like the VFW, born in the Vietnam era, largely fail to resonate with modern veterans. Many find these spaces too formal, overly focused on alcohol, or unwelcoming to families. Today's veterans often seek more family-friendly, wellness-oriented communities that foster connections and support personal growth.

Psychedelic healing naturally encourages community building. Group sessions help veterans recognize the importance of authentic connection, vulnerability, and mutual support. They create spaces where veterans can share their unique experiences, including gallows humor and shared understanding of military life, while developing deeper, more meaningful relationships than typically possible in civilian settings.

This is why HHP prioritizes group retreats followed by ongoing integration circles. As veterans complete their initial psychedelic experiences, they join existing communities of veterans supporting each other through the integration process. These groups evolve organically as new members join, creating sustainable support networks that help veterans stay accountable to their healing journey.

While online connections and virtual meetings serve a purpose, they cannot replace the human need for in-person community. In an era of increasing digital isolation, veteran healing communities fill a vital role: providing spaces for authentic connection, mutual support, and shared growth.

This is the vision of HHP for all veterans, not just the ones who do psychedelics. While psychedelic experiences can catalyze deeper connections and vulnerability, the human need for community transcends any particular healing modality. Veterans need spaces where they can be fully themselves, where their military identity is honored rather than pathologized, and where they can build meaningful connections.

WHAT'S NEXT?

Your healing journey doesn't end with this book. It's just the beginning.

Heroic Hearts Project connects veterans with leading medical researchers and pioneering psychedelic treatment programs designed specifically for service-related trauma. Whether you're exploring your options, ready to take action, or supporting a veteran in your life, we have pathways forward.

Visit **heroicheartsproject.org** to:

- Explore veteran-centered psychedelic programs and retreats
- Read stories from veterans who've found healing
- Apply for treatment or learn about next steps
- Support this lifesaving work with a donation

One final mission: Leave a review of this book on Amazon or your preferred bookseller.

Every review reaches more veterans who need to know that healing is possible. Your voice matters. Please help us get this information into the hands of those who need it most.

BIBLIOGRAPHY

Aloi, J. A. (2011). A theoretical study of the hidden wounds of war: Disenfranchised grief and the impact on nursing practice. *ISRN Nursing, 2011*, 716479.

America's Warrior Partnership. (2022). *Operation Deep Dive: Summary of Interim Report*. America's Warrior Partnership. Retrieved from https://www.americaswarriorpartnership.org/opdd-archives

Audacy. (2018, September 11). How many troops are dying in training accidents and why? Connecting Vets.

Blest-Hopley, G., Pasculli, G., Ruffell, S. G. D., Tsang, W., Emmanuel, O., Pate, K. M., Kettner, H., Roseman, L., Erritzoe, D., & Carhart-Harris, R. (2025). Improved mental health outcomes and normalised spontaneous EEG activity in veterans reporting a history of traumatic brain injuries following participation in a psilocybin retreat. *Frontiers in Psychiatry, 16*, 1594307.

Calnan, M., Blest-Hopley, G., Busch, C., Adams, M., Ruffell, S. G. D., Piper, T., Roseman, L., Kettner, H., & Carhart-Harris, R. (2025). Exploring the therapeutic effects of psychedelics administered to military veterans in naturalistic retreat settings. *Brain and Behavior, 15*(7), e70660.

Carhart-Harris, R. L., Bolstridge, M., Rucker, J., Day, C. M. J., Erritzoe, D., Kaelen, M., Bloomfield, M., Rickard, J. A., Forbes, B., Feilding, A., Taylor, D., Pilling, S., Curran, V. H., & Nutt, D. J. (2016). Psilocybin with psychological support for treatment-resistant depression: An open-label feasibility study. *The Lancet Psychiatry, 3*(7), 619–627.

Carhart-Harris, R. L., & Goodwin, G. M. (2017). The therapeutic potential of psychedelic drugs: Past, present, and future. *Neuropsychopharmacology, 42*(11), 2105–2113.

Carhart-Harris, R. L., Bolstridge, M., Day, C. M. J., Rucker, J., Watts, R., Erritzoe, D. E., Kaelen, M., Giribaldi, B., Bloomfield, M., Pilling, S., Rickard, J. A., Forbes, B., Feilding, A., Taylor, D., Curran, H. V., & Nutt, D. J. (2018). Psilocybin with psychological support for treatment-resistant depression: Six-month follow-up. *Psychopharmacology, 235*(2), 399–408.

Conti, P. (2022). *Trauma: The invisible epidemic: How trauma works and how we can heal from it*. St. Martin's Press.

Davis, A. K., Clifton, J. M., Weaver, E. G., Hurwitz, E. S., Johnson, M. W., & Griffiths, R. R. (2020). Survey of 5-MeO-DMT use: Epidemiology, motivations, and acute subjective effects. Journal of Psychedelic Studies, 4(1), 1–10.

Davis, A. K., So, S., Lancelotta, R., Barsuglia, J. P., & Griffiths, R. R. (2019). 5-MeO-DMT used in a naturalistic group setting is associated with unintended improvements in depression and anxiety. The American Journal of Drug and Alcohol Abuse, 45(2), 161–169.

Dworkin, E. R., Ullman, S. E., Stappenbeck, C., Brill, C. D., & Kaysen, D. (2018). Proximal relationships between social support and PTSD symptom severity: A daily diary study of sexual assault survivors. *Depression and anxiety*, *35*(1), 43–49.

Fares-Otero, N. E., Sharp, T. H., Balle, S. R., Quaatz, S. M., Vieta, E., Åhs, F., Allgaier, A. K., Arévalo, A., Bachem, R., Belete, H., Mossie, T. B., Berzengi, A., Capraz, N., Ceylan, D., Dukes, D., Essadek, A., Iqbal, N., Jobson, L., Levy-Gigi, E., Lüönd, A., Halligan, S. L. (2024). Social support and (complex) posttraumatic stress symptom severity: does gender matter?. *European journal of psychotraumatology*, *15*(1), 2398921.

Griffiths, R. R., Johnson, M. W., Carducci, M. A., Umbricht, A., Richards, W. A., Richards, B. D., Cosimano, M. P., & Klinedinst, M. A. (2016). Psilocybin produces substantial and sustained decreases in depression and anxiety in patients with life-threatening cancer: A randomized double-blind trial. *Journal of Psychopharmacology*, *30*(12), 1181–1197.

Hogan, N. J. (2024). Martial Culture in the Lifeways of US Servicemembers and Veterans: Military Psychology, Ancient Mythology, and Re-Souling Service. Routledge.

Institute of Medicine. (2009). Gulf War and Health, Volume 7: Long-Term Consequences of Traumatic Brain Injury. Washington, DC: The National Academies Press.

Junger, S. (2016). *Tribe: On homecoming and belonging.* HarperCollins.

Kato K, Kleinhenz JM, Shin YJ, Coarfa C, Zarrabi AJ, Hecker L. Psilocybin treatment extends cellular lifespan and improves survival of aged mice. NPJ Aging. 2025 Jul 8;11(1):55. doi: 10.1038/s41514-025-00244-x. PMID: 40628762; PMCID: PMC12238350.

Kelley, M. L., Bravo, A. J., Hamrick, H. C., Braitman, A. L., & Judah, M. R. (2019). Killing during combat and negative mental health and substance use outcomes among recent-era veterans: The mediating effects of rumination. Psychological Trauma: Theory, Research, Practice, and Policy, 11(4), 379–382.

Kilner, P. (2002, March–April). Military leaders' obligation to justify killing in war. *Military Review, 82*(2), 24–31.

Kittel, J. A., Monteith, L. L., Holliday, R., Morano, T. T., Schneider, A. L., Brenner, L. A., & Hoffmire, C. A. (2025). *Geospatial estimates of suicidal ideation and suicide attempt prevalence in the U.S. veteran population (2022). Injury Epidemiology, 12,* Article 32.

Miller, L. (2025, June 17). *Statistics on veterans and substance abuse.* Veteran Addiction.

Mitchell, J. M., Bogenschutz, M., Lilienstein, A., Harrison, C., Kleiman, S., Parker-Guilbert, K., Ot'alora, G. M., Garas, W., Paleos, C., Gorman, I., Nicholas, C. R., Mithoefer, M. C., Carlin, S., Poulter, B., Mithoefer, A., Quevedo, S., Wells, G., Klaire, S. S., van der Kolk, B., … Doblin, R. (2021). MDMA-assisted therapy for severe PTSD: A randomized, double-blind, placebo-controlled phase 3 study. *Nature Medicine, 27*(6), 1025–1033.

Mithoefer, M. C., Feduccia, A. A., Jerome, L., Wagner, M., Wymer, J., Hamilton, S., Yazar-Klosinski, B., Emerson, A., & Doblin, R. (2018). MDMA-assisted psychotherapy for treatment of PTSD: Long-term follow-up of a randomized controlled trial. *Journal of Psychopharmacology, 32*(1), 28–40.

Mithoefer, M. C., Wagner, M. T., Mithoefer, A. T., Jerome, L., & Doblin, R. (2013). Durability of improvement in post-traumatic stress disorder symptoms and absence of harmful effects or drug dependency after 3,4-methylenedioxymethamphetamine-assisted psychotherapy: A prospective long-term follow-up study. *Journal of Psychopharmacology, 27*(1), 28–39.

Moore MJ, Shawler E, Jordan CH, et al. Veteran and Military Mental Health Issues. [Updated 2023 Aug 17]. In: StatPearls [Internet]. Treasure Island (FL): StatPearls Publishing; 2025 Jan.

Nathanson, D. L. (1998). Affect Theory and the Compass of Shame. In The Widening Scope of Shame (pp. 16-). Routledge.

National Institute on Drug Abuse. (2020, March). Substance use and military life. National Institutes of Health.

Ngo, T. P., Keyhani, S., Leonard, S., & Hoggatt, K. J. (2025). Substance use and use disorders among Veterans on long-term opioid therapy. *Drug and alcohol dependence reports*, *16*, 100347.

Norrholm, S. D., Maples-Keller, J. L., Rothbaum, B. O., & Tossell, C. C. (2020). Remote warfare with intimate consequences: Psychological stress in service member and veteran remotely-piloted aircraft (RPA) personnel. Journal of Mental Health and Clinical Psychology, 4(4), 10–17.

Ot'alora, G. M., Grigsby, J., Poulter, B., Van Derveer, J. W., Giron, S. G., Jerome, L., Feduccia, A. A., Hamilton, S., Yazar-Klosinski, B., Emerson, A., & Mithoefer, M. C. (2018). 3,4-Methylenedioxymethamphetamine-assisted psychotherapy for treatment of chronic posttraumatic stress disorder: A randomized phase 2 controlled trial. *Journal of Psychopharmacology, 32*(12), 1295–1307.

Palmer, C., Ferber, A. T., & Greenwald, B. D. (2025). The potential role of psilocybin in traumatic brain injury recovery: A narrative review. *Brain Sciences, 15*(6), 572.

Pew Research Center. (2011, November 8). For many injured veterans, a lifetime of consequences. Pew Research Center's Social & Demographic Trends.

Raut, S., Mellor, R., Meurk, C., Lam, M., Lane, J., Khoo, A., Cronin, A., Smith, S., Heffernan, E., & Johnson, L. (2025). Prevalence and factors associated with polypharmacy in military and veteran populations: A systematic review and meta-analysis. Journal of Affective Disorders, 369, 411–420.

Ross, S., Bossis, A., Guss, J., Agin-Liebes, G., Malone, T., Cohen, B., Mennenga, S. E., Belser, A., Kalliontzi, K., Babb, J., Su, Z., Corby, P., & Schmidt, B. L. (2016). Rapid and sustained symptom reduction following psilocybin treatment for anxiety and depression in patients with life-threatening cancer: A randomized controlled trial. *Journal of Psychopharmacology, 30*(12), 1165–1180.

Rossi, F. S., Nillni, Y. I., Fox, A. B., Galovski, T. E., & [additional authors]. (2025). Gender and ethnoracial disparities in veterans' trauma exposure prevalence across life phases. *Injury Epidemiology.* Advance online publication.

Ruiz, F., Burgo-Black, L., Hunt, S. C., Miller, M., & Spelman, J. F. (2023). A practical review of suicide among veterans: Preventive and proactive measures for health care institutions and providers. *Public Health Reports, 138*(2), 223–231.

Saini, R. K., V K Raju, M. S., & Chail, A. (2021). Cry in the sky: Psychological impact on drone operators. *Industrial psychiatry journal, 30*(Suppl 1), S15–S19. https://doi.org/10.4103/0972-6748.328782

Sessa, B. (2017). MDMA and PTSD treatment: "PTSD: From novel pathophysiology to innovative therapeutics." *Progress in Neuro-Psychopharmacology & Biological Psychiatry, 84,* 220–228.

Stein, M. B., Ipser, J. C., & Seedat, S. (2006). Pharmacotherapy for posttraumatic stress disorder: A systematic review and meta-analysis. *JAMA, 296*(5), 637–650.

Suitt, T. H. (2021, June 21). High suicide rates among United States service members and veterans of the post-9/11 wars. Costs of War Project, Watson Institute for International and Public Affairs, Brown University.

Tokar, S. (2010, February 10). Killing in Iraq combat linked with PTSD, alcohol abuse, other problems. UCSF News Center.

U.S. Department of Veterans Affairs. (n.d.). *Coping with grief.* Whole Health Library. https://www.va.gov/WHOLEHEALTHLIBRARY/overviews/coping-with-grief.asp

U.S. Department of Veterans Affairs. (2025). How common is PTSD among Veterans and among civilians? National Center for PTSD.

U.S. Department of Veterans Affairs. (n.d.). Military sexual trauma (MST). National Center for PTSD.

U.S. Department of Veterans Affairs. (2024). 2024 National Veteran Suicide Prevention Annual Report (Part 2 of 2). Office of Mental Health and Suicide Prevention.

Uthaug, M. V., Davis, A. K., Haas, T. F., Davis, D., Dolan, S. B., Lancelotta, R., … & Ramaekers, J. G. (2019). A single inhalation of vapor from dried toad secretion containing 5-MeO-DMT in a naturalistic setting is associated with sustained enhancement of satisfaction with life, mindfulness-related capacities, and a decrement of psychopathological symptoms. Psychopharmacology, 236(9), 2653–2666.

Velit-Salazar, M. R., Shiroma, P. R., & Cherian, E. (2024). A systematic review of the neurocognitive effects of psychedelics in healthy populations: Implications for depressive disorders and post-traumatic stress disorder. *Brain Sciences*, *14*(3), 248.

Wong, L., & Gerras, S. J. (2015). Lying to ourselves: Dishonesty in the Army profession. U.S. Army War College Strategic Studies Institute.

Yasin, B., Mehta, S., Tewfik, G., & Bekker, A. (2024). Psychedelics as novel therapeutic agents for chronic pain. Mechanisms and future perspectives. *Explorations in Neuroscience, 3,* 418–433.

ACKNOWLEDGEMENTS

From Jesse:

To the veterans who've served and continue to serve: your courage and sacrifice built the foundation on which this work stands.

To the brothers and sisters who shared your time, stories, and experience to shape this project: thank you for your generosity, your vulnerability, and for carrying the torch forward.

To those who have stepped into the unknown, participating in research and early programs: your willingness to lead from the front has opened doors for countless others.

To every veteran who has stood at the forefront of mental health, demanding better solutions: you remind us that this fight is not over, that the veteran voice matters, and that healing is a mission worth pursuing together.

To the volunteers, supporters, and professionals who stand beside our community, advocating, educating, and helping to expand access to care: your dedication ensures that this movement continues to grow with integrity and heart.

This manual is for you, because of you, and dedicated to all who continue the work of service, both on the battlefield and within.

From Elaine:

First, thanks to Jesse Gould for taking a chance on an unknown for this collaboration. It was richly rewarding, and I hope it helps further the cause.

I want to thank the veterans and first responders, those who support their healing, and their partners who spoke with vulnerability and candor about their experiences and helped educate this clueless civilian: Lauren Connally, Tim Foxley, Jamie Fremgen, Josh Gage, Angela Graham, Nathan Hogan, PhD, Tim Houweling, Samantha Juan, Jason Lane, Tambi Lane, Mark Keller, Bob Kaufmann, MD, Anthony Longo, Chris Maddox, Nathaniel Mills, PhD, LCP, Patrick Mullins, Jared Reinhart, Alex Robinson, Zach Skiles, PsyD, Will Tovar, Colin Wells, Allison Wilson, Tommy Wisdom, Carl Bonnett, MD, Chris, and Dave.

Special thanks to Nathan Hogan, PhD, for your great work on exploring martial culture.

Thanks to Swel Myat Sandi Min Thein for helping keep many plates spinning, Hannah Kimyon for organizational support, and Steven Hall, Barry Callen, and Melanie Balsis for the excellent design and illustration work. Thanks to Benjamin Kelley of Relevāre for book production.

Lastly, thanks to all the veterans and first responders for stepping into service in a culture where your sacrifices go largely unseen. My biggest hope is that this book helps you feel seen, validated, and valued, and perhaps even offers a path out of darkness.

www.ingramcontent.com/pod-product-compliance
Lightning Source LLC
Chambersburg PA
CBHW051621120626
46551CB00014B/1895